Chi Nei Ching

Chi Nei Ching

Muscle, Tendon, and Meridian Massage

Mantak Chia and
William U. Wei

Destiny Books
Rochester, Vermont • Toronto, Canada

Destiny Books
One Park Street
Rochester, Vermont 05767
www.DestinyBooks.com

Destiny Books is a division of Inner Traditions International

Originally published in Thailand in 2012 by Universal Tao Publications under the title *Chi Nei Ching: Internal Muscle, Tendon, Meridian Massage*

Library of Congress Cataloging-in-Publication Data
Chia, Mantak, 1944–
  Chi nei ching : muscle, tendon, and meridian massage / Mantak Chia and William U. Wei.
      pages cm
  Other title: Chi nei tsang III
  Includes index.
  ISBN 978-1-62055-086-1 (pbk.) — ISBN 978-1-62055-133-2 (e-book)
  1. Qi gong. 2. Tai chi. 3. Massage therapy. I. Wei, William U. II. Title. III. Title: Chi nei tsang III.
  RM727.C54C448 2013
  613.7'1489—dc23
                                                                                    2012051318

Printed and bound in the United States by Versa Press, Inc.

10 9 8 7 6 5 4 3 2 1

Text design and layout by Priscilla Baker
This book was typeset in Janson with Sho, Futura, Diotima, and Present used as display typefaces
Illustrations by Udon Jandee
Photographs by Sopitnapa Promnon

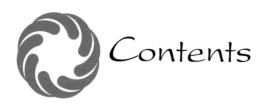

Contents

Acknowledgments   vii

Putting Chi Nei Ching into Practice   ix

Introduction: The Concepts of Chi Nei Ching   1

PART ONE

Eastern and Western Anatomy for Chi Nei Ching Practitioners

1 ● Western Medical Anatomy: The Muscles and Tendons   6

2 ● Thai Medical Anatomy: The Sen Lines   16

3 ● Chinese Medical Anatomy:
The Tendinomuscular Meridians   30

PART TWO

Treating the Muscles, Tendons, and Meridians with Chi Nei Ching

4 ● Preparing for Chi Nei Ching Practice   46

5 ● Nuad Thai: Thai Therapeutic Massage   58

6 ● Traditional Tok Sen   110

7 ● Meridian Detoxification Therapy   154

About the Authors   171

The Universal Healing Tao System and Training Center   173

Index   175

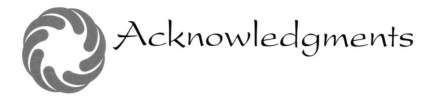

Acknowledgments

The Universal Tao publications staff involved in the preparation and production of *Chi Nei Ching* extend our gratitude to the many generations of Taoist Masters who have passed on their special lineage, in the form of an unbroken oral transmission, over thousands of years. We thank Taoist Master I Yun Yi Eng for his openness in transmitting the formulas of Taoist Inner Alchemy.

We also wish to thank the Chi Nei Tsang teacher Dr. Mui Yimwattana, who has worked so patiently to teach his students. Special thanks to Intorn Hoykaew for understanding and teaching the Tok Sen techniques.

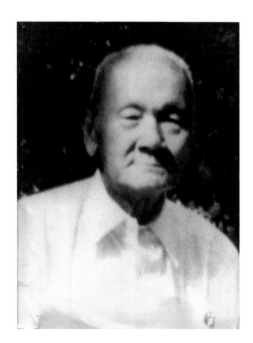

Master Mui Yimwattana

We offer our eternal gratitude and love to our parents and teachers for their many gifts to us. Remembering them brings joy and satisfaction to our continued efforts in presenting the Universal Healing Tao system. As always, their contribution has been crucial in presenting the concepts and techniques of the Universal Healing Tao. We also wish to thank the thousands of unknown men and women of the Taoist healing arts who developed many of the methods and ideas presented in this book.

Special thanks to Koravee Tharnpipat for translating portions of the text from Thai into English.

We thank the many contributors essential to this book's final form: the editorial and production staff at Inner Traditions/Destiny Books for their efforts to clarify the text and produce a handsome new edition of the book, Nancy Yeilding for her developmental edit, and Gail Rex for her line edit of the new edition.

For their efforts on the first edition of this book, we thank our Thai production team: Hirunyathorn Punsan, Sopitnapa Promnon, Udon Jandee, and Suthisa Chaisam.

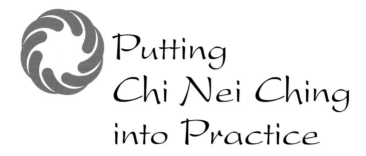

Putting Chi Nei Ching into Practice

The information presented in this book is based on the authors' personal experience and knowledge of Taoist healing and practices. The practices described in this book have been used successfully for thousands of years by Taoists trained by personal instruction. Readers should not undertake the practices without receiving personal transmission and training from a certified instructor of the Universal Healing Tao, since certain of these practices, if done improperly, may cause injury or result in health problems. This book is intended to supplement individual training by the Universal Healing Tao and to serve as a reference guide for these practices. Anyone who undertakes these practices on the basis of this book alone, does so entirely at his or her own risk.

The meditations, practices, and techniques described herein are not intended to be used as an alternative or substitute for professional medical treatment and care. If any readers are suffering from illnesses based on mental or emotional disorders, an appropriate professional health care practitioner or therapist should be consulted. Such problems should be corrected before you start training.

Neither the Universal Healing Tao nor its staff and instructors can be responsible for the consequences of any practice or misuse of the information contained in this book. If the reader undertakes any exercise without strictly following the instructions, notes, and warnings, the responsibility must lie solely with the reader.

This book does not attempt to give any medical diagnosis, treatment, prescription, or remedial recommendation in relation to any human disease, ailment, suffering, or physical condition whatsoever.

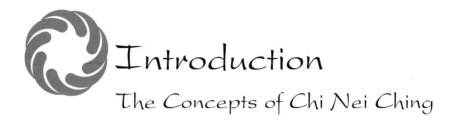

Introduction

The Concepts of Chi Nei Ching

Chi Nei Ching is the fourth and final book in the Chi Nei Tsang series, which focuses on massage techniques that move energy (chi) throughout the body while releasing and opening up its passages. The first three books in the series—*Chi Nei Tsang, Advanced Chi Nei Tsang,* and *Karsai Nei Tsang*—focus on organs and meridians deep within the body, while this volume focuses on the meridians, muscles, and tendons that are closer to the body's surface. The goal of Chi Nei Ching is to improve the flow of chi in these tissues in order to eliminate health problems and improve the overall quality of life.

The concepts and practices of Chi Nei Ching represent the long history of interaction between the medical traditions of China, India, and Thailand. The approaches to health and well-being included here date back many centuries; the concept of chi is at least twenty-five centuries old and traditional Asian medicine at least twenty-two centuries old. This volume is the first to focus intensively on traditional Thai medicine's contributions to the Universal Healing Tao practices.

Every aspect and part of the human body is discussed either directly or indirectly in this book. That is because the Thai approach, unlike Western medicine, is much more holistic. Nothing can be treated or discussed in isolation. Rather it must be seen as part of an organic whole that is related to, influences, and is influenced by every other part of the body.

Part 1 of this book details the particulars of Eastern and Western anatomy that Chi Nei Ching practitioners rely on when administering tendon massage or other techniques. While Western anatomy maps the physical structures of tendon, muscle, and connective tissue, it is the Thai anatomy of Sen lines and the Chinese tendinomuscular meridians that relate these structures to specific signs of health and dysfunction. It is these lines and meridians that allow the skilled practitioner to turn a muscle massage into a medical treatment. Everyone, even those with just a passing interest in traditional Thai approaches to health and longevity, should have an idea of what these meridians are and how they function. Such an understanding can improve knowledge of one's body, which is essential for maintaining energy, well-being, and overall quality of life.

Part 2 explores the practices that address the tendons and muscles specifically. Chapter 4 reviews the ways that a practitioner should prepare him- or herself for working with a student. Chapter 5 details the practice of Thai therapeutic massage—the aspect of Thai holistic health care and maintenance that clears blockages from the tendons to facilitate healing and freedom of movement. From the arms and hands to the lower extremities and the trunk, Thai massage therapy facilitates improved vitality, using healing techniques that have been practiced and proven effective in Thailand for centuries.

Chapter 6 examines the unique Thai practice of Tok Sen, which uses a wooden hammer and a variety of wooden pegs known as *pestles* to gently tap the tissues and tendons into balance. One of the most important contributions to traditional healing in Asia, Tok Sen has its roots in Chiang Mai, Thailand. It dates back thousands of years and is a key part of the Lanna culture of the region. The primary function of Tok Sen is to treat pain issues relating to the tendons and muscles.

Chapter 7, the final chapter of the book, focuses on meridian detoxification therapy, particularly through cupping and Gua Sha, two powerful techniques that release built-up toxins from the subcutaneous tissues. The latter is dealt with in detail and includes many illustrations in addition to a discussion of the fundamental method of applying this effective folk treatment to different parts of the anatomy.

The overall purpose of this book is to present alternative treatments for illness as well as methods of health maintenance; these are intended to help our readers experience a healthy and energetic life. While some of the treatments, such as massage therapy, are somewhat familiar in the West, others, like Tok Sen and Gua Sha, are little known. Frequently a combination of treatments complements one another and amplifies the benefits of the therapy. Anyone interested in health, well-being, and longevity will benefit from this unique book.

PART 1

Eastern and Western Anatomy for Chi Nei Ching Practitioners

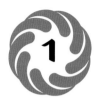

Western Medical Anatomy

The Muscles and Tendons

A general understanding of human anatomy is important for the Chi Nei Ching practitioner. It is not necessary to know the name of every muscle, bone, tendon, and ligament, but understanding the ways that the body connects to itself is important. Furthermore, the practitioner who is familiar with the structure of the body will be more proficient and more "connected" to the individual receiving treatment.

MUSCLES

Skeletal muscles consist of bundles of muscle fibers, called *fascicles*, that are wrapped in fibrous connective tissue and supplied with blood (fig. 1.1). Bundles of such fascicles wrapped together form the belly of each individual muscle.

It is helpful to know the names and locations of significant muscle groups. Figures 1.2 and 1.3 on pages 8 and 9 show some of the more important muscles from lateral, front, and rear views.

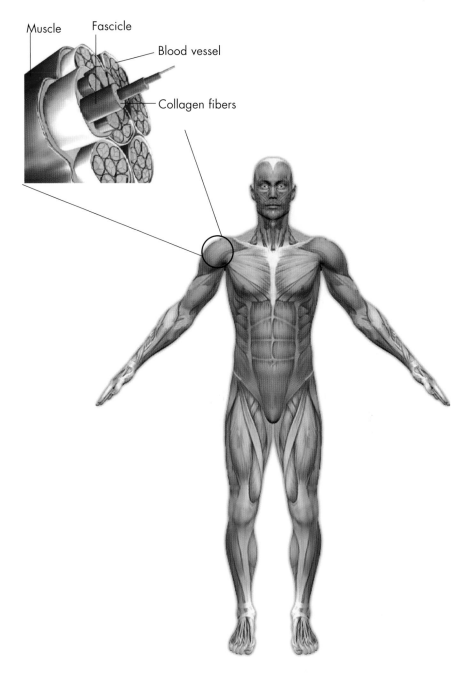

Muscle   Fascicle

Blood vessel

Collagen fibers

Fig. 1.1. Muscles are composed of bundles of muscle
fibers wrapped together in connective tissue.

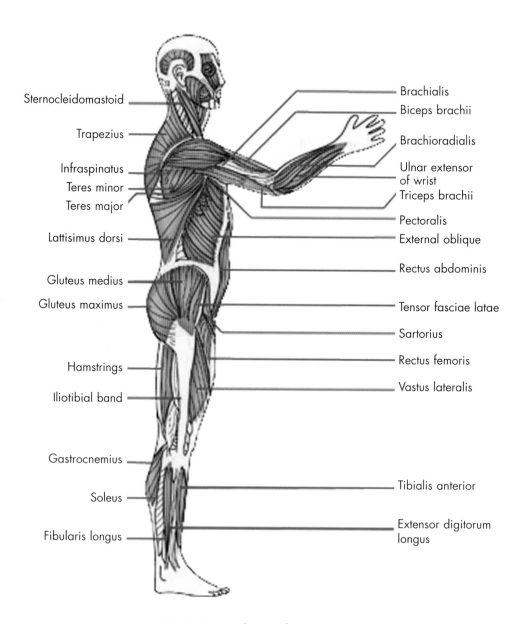

Sternocleidomastoid

Trapezius

Infraspinatus

Teres minor

Teres major

Lattisimus dorsi

Gluteus medius

Gluteus maximus

Hamstrings

Iliotibial band

Gastrocnemius

Soleus

Fibularis longus

Brachialis

Biceps brachii

Brachioradialis

Ulnar extensor of wrist

Triceps brachii

Pectoralis

External oblique

Rectus abdominis

Tensor fasciae latae

Sartorius

Rectus femoris

Vastus lateralis

Tibialis anterior

Extensor digitorum longus

Fig. 1.2. Lateral view of major muscles

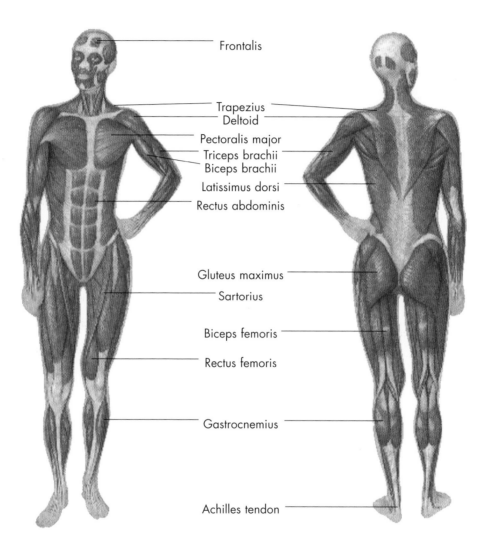

Fig. 1.3. Front and rear view of major muscles

TENDONS

Tendons are found throughout the body, occurring wherever the muscles connect to the bones (fig. 1.4). They support the movement and structure of the body by providing stability and flexibility. Tendons are composed of fibrous connective tissue. This tissue is arranged in dense, regular bundles of fibers that give tremendous strength while still maintaining pliancy.

In a well-maintained and healthy human body, tendons are flexible and can be compared to rubber bands. Working with the muscles as they stretch, tendons exert a pulling force. Numerous injuries are possible with the tendons, including pulls, tears, and inflammatory conditions like tendonitis. These can result from many sources including, for example, age, body weight, and strain.

There are around four thousand tendons in the human body, but the number can vary. Tendons run mostly up and down with some, for example, extending from the neck all the way down through the toes.

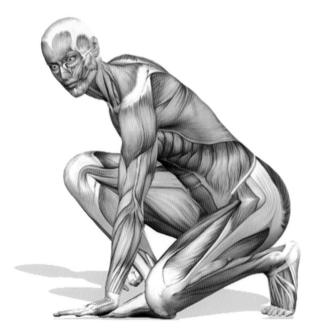

Fig. 1.4. Tendons are tough bands of fibrous connective tissue.

While it is not necessary to know the precise location of thousands of tendons, it is possible to check for problems by touching and viewing the areas where treatment is needed.

Practitioners can evaluate the condition of the muscles and tendons as a part of a basic assessment of the client's body. The important thing to know is how to apply resistance against a muscle as you palpate along it to discover where any problems might reside. To evaluate the muscles and tendons of the upper leg, for example, the practitioner can ask the client to lie down on her back and rotate one bent leg inward. The therapist applies resistance to this inward push while palpating the tendons and muscles of the upper leg for issues. Generally, problems areas are evident because they are "armored" or hard. Often they are painful if pressure is applied to them, especially while meeting resistance.

LIGAMENTS AND FASCIA

Like the tendons, ligaments and fascia are also composed of collagen fibers, but ligaments join one bone to another bone, and fascia connects muscles to organs and other muscles, whereas tendons exclusively connect muscles to bones. Ligaments restrain the movement of bones at a joint and are therefore important in preventing dislocation. Ligaments also support various organs, including the uterus, bladder, liver, and diaphragm, and they help to maintain the shape of the breasts. It should be noted that in some cases ligaments are gender specific, helping to support the uterus in women, for example.

Fascia is a sheet or band of fibrous tissue separating or binding muscles and organs in the body. In fact, fascia is the tissue that connects all parts of the body, surrounding and connecting each nerve, bone, muscle, tendon, and organ. A healthy fascial system is flexible. If fascia is tight or rigid, pain and stiffness can result—not just in the region of tightness, but also in other areas that may be compensating for this rigidity. The fascial system, like everything, needs to be maintained for the body to be healthy.

In Eastern medicine, fascia is a structure for and a conduit of chi. The meridians and channels pass through fascia, keeping the tissue moist and dense with chi. When the chi is deficient, fascia becomes dry, hard, and brittle; movement can become painful. Chi Nei Ching practices are designed to free up the fascia and help it be a better conduit of chi.

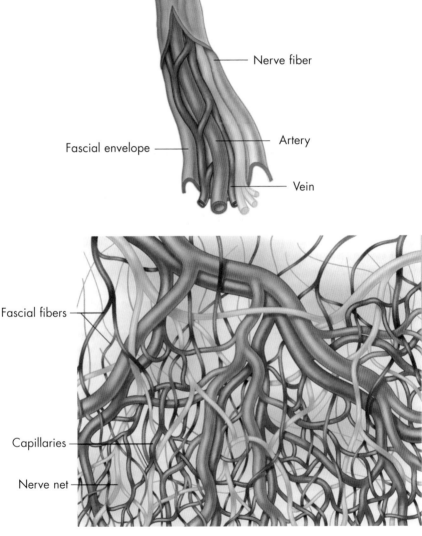

Fig. 1.5. Neural, vascular, and fascial systems

NERVES AND BLOOD VESSELS

Like the fascial system, the neural system also connects different parts of the body to each other, but whereas the fascia connects via fibers and tissues, the nervous system sends electrical and chemical signals between different parts of the body via the neurons. A close examination of the nervous system reveals that it spreads out like the roots of a tree: the nerves get smaller and smaller as they stretch from the spinal cord out to the extremities (fig 1.5).

The circulatory system is made up of arteries and veins, with the arteries carrying oxygen-rich blood from the heart to the rest of the body, and the veins returning oxygen-poor blood back to the heart. The heart itself is tendon-like and fibrous in its construction. The circulatory system, like other systems of the body, can become stiff— particularly with age. Keeping it healthy and flexible is vital to the continuation of good health in our later years.

This complex arrangement of tubes and fibers can get tangled, causing pain, impaired mobility, or dysfunction. If these problems continue unchecked, they may lead to greater health problems.

THE SPINE

Because of the spine's intimate relationship with the nervous system and the entire skeleton, its health influences almost everything in the body. Many problems in the body can originate in the spine, though this origin is not always immediately evident. It is possible, for example, that a problem in the spine can be the cause of headaches, leg pain, arm numbness, sleep issues, etc. A thorough knowledge of the spine and its relationship—via the nerves—to the rest of the body is thus extremely useful to a therapist in addressing most health problems.

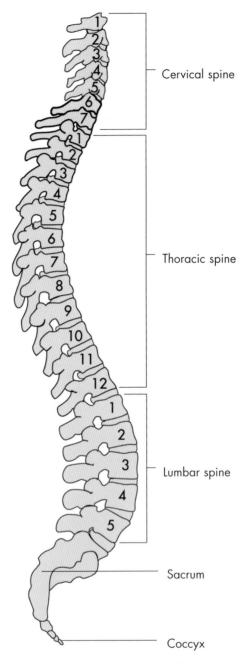

Cervical spine

Thoracic spine

Lumbar spine

Sacrum

Coccyx

Fig. 1.6. The sections of the spine

Spinal Alignment

The alignment of the spine can be checked visually as well as by palpating: most people have two "dimples" at the lower part of the spine just above the buttock. These should be horizontally even—essentially opposite from each other across the spine. If they are not, then they need to be realigned.

 ## Simple Spinal Alignment

1. Determine which leg has the higher dimple above it. Ask the client to stand on something, say a thick book, while letting the leg with the higher dimple drop down.
2. Have the client swing the dropped leg gently back and forth. At the same time, apply pressure with the palm of your hand to the dimple.
3. Then check the dimples again.

This technique is effective in many instances of lower back pain as well other back issues.

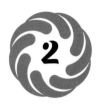

Thai Medical Anatomy
The Sen Lines

The distinct styles of medicine that arose in the Far East developed systems of anatomy that focused on the movement of energy through the body, rather than on the physical anatomical tissues exclusively. In Thai medicine, the Sen lines map the ways that energy moves through the body (fig. 2.1).

The ten energy lines known as the Sen Sib are part of a system of medicine that is thought to be thousands of years old. The ancient *Royal Traditional Thai Medicine Text* describes seventy-two thousand channels, which are organized along the ten main lines of the Sen Sib. These channels spread out from the abdominal cavity carrying chi or energy throughout the body. A unique and special feature of Thai medicine, the Sen Sib have been the heart of Thai massage throughout the history of Thailand.

Although therapeutic Thai massage is unique to Thailand, its concepts originated from India and China, and the ten "wind" channels are related to those found in Chinese medicine. While the overall philosophy underlying the different schools of Chinese, Indian, and Thai massage is fundamentally the same, the names and numbers of

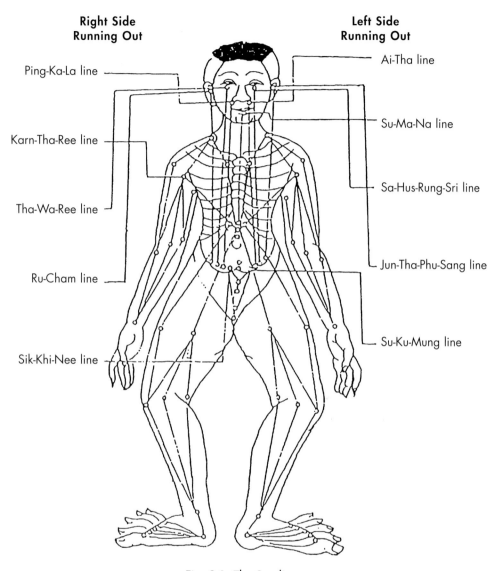

Fig. 2.1. The Sen lines

the lines differ across the traditions, as do the specifics of massage practice.

Almost all of the ancient textbooks describing the details of Thai medicine were destroyed during repeated invasions of the region; by the early nineteenth century, these ancient practices were in danger of being lost entirely. In 1832, King Rama III ordered all of the known medical teachings to be inscribed into the stone walls of the royal monastery in Bangkok, so that they would be effectively preserved. Known as the Wat Pho plaques, these carvings depict sixty energy channels in the body—thirty on the front and thirty on the back, along with treatment protocols for specific points on these channels.

THE NAMES OF THE TEN ENERGY CHANNELS

While the few surviving ancient texts show that the ten main channels have been known by a variety of names throughout history, this book will use the names that are most common today. The table below shows some variant names for the Sen Sib, as they appear in texts compiled in the nineteenth century. Among these were the *Royal Traditional Thai Medicine Text*, gathered in the era of King Rama V (around 1880); the *Tamla Loke Nitan* (medicinal fables) from the reign of King Rama II (1809–1824); and the Wat Pho tab-

HISTORICAL NAMES OF SEN SIB

SEN SIB NUMBER	SEN SIB NAME/ ROYAL MEDICINE TEXT	SEN SIB NAME/ TAMLA LOKE NITAN	SEN SIB NAME/ WAT PHO EPIGRAPHS
1	I-Tha	I-Tha	I-Tha
2	Ping-Kla	Ping-Kla	Ping-Kla
3	Sum-Ma-Na	Sum-Ma-Na	Sum-Ma-Na
4	Kan-La-Ta-Ree	Kan-La-Ta-Ree	Kan-La-Ta-Ree
5	Sa-Had-Sa-Rang-Sri	Sa-Had-Sa-Rang-Sri	Sa-Had-Sa-Rang-Sri
6	Ta-Wa-Ree	Ta-Wa-Ka-Ta	Ta-Wa-Ree
7	La-Wu-Sank	U-Rang	Jan-Ta-Pu-Sank
8	U-Lang-Ga	Su-Kum-U-Sa-Ma	Ru-Sum
9	Ta-Wa-Tha-Ree	Kang-Ku	Su-Ku-Mang
10	Sik-Ki-Nee	Sank-Ki-Nee	Si-Ki-Nee

lets described above, recorded during the reign of King Rama III (1824–1851).

In this book, we will refer to the ten Sen Sib using the names in most common current use:

1. Itha
2. Pingkla
3. Summana
4. Kanlataree
5. Hadsarangsri
6. Tawaree
7. Jantapusank
8. Rusum
9. Sukumang
10. Sikinee

DESCRIPTIONS OF THE SEN SIB

All of the ten channels start near the abdomen, a region that is extremely important in traditional Thai therapy, as it is in Chi Nei Tsang and traditional Chinese medicine. While all ten Sen lines start roughly in the area of the navel, each follows a different course through the body.

Sen 1: Itha

Left Side of the Body, Exits Left Nostril

Itha begins one thumb-width to the left side of the navel and passes through the pubic area to the back of the left thigh (see fig. 2.2 on page 20). It then runs upward past the left buttock and proceeds along the left side of spine, continuing over the head and curving downward to the left side of the face, and exiting from the left nostril.

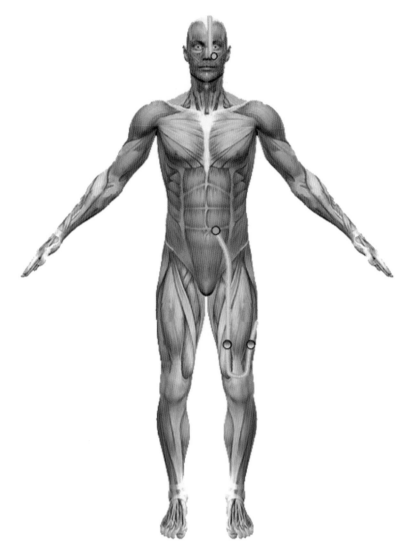

Fig. 2.2. The Itha line

Conditions: Headache, stiff neck, shoulder pain, common cold, cough, nasal obstruction, sore throat, eye pain, chill and fever, abdominal pain, intestinal diseases, back pain, diseases of the urinary tract, dizziness.

Sen 2: Pingkla

Right Side of the Body, Exits Right Nostril

Pingkla begins one thumb-width to the right side of the navel and passes through the pubic area to the back of the right thigh. It then runs upward past the right buttock and proceeds along the right side of spine, continuing over the head and curving downward to the right side of the face to exit from the right nostril (fig. 2.3).

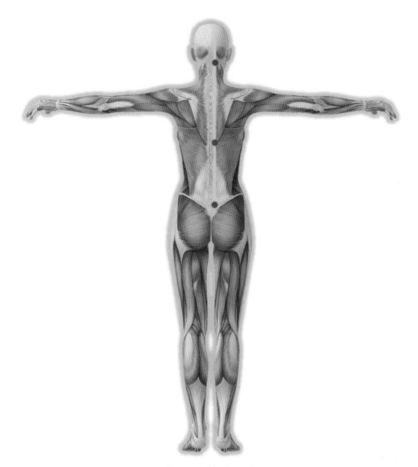

Fig. 2.3. The Pingkla line, back side

Conditions: Same as Sen Itha. Additional indications: diseases of the liver and the gallbladder.

Sen 3: Summana

Front Midline of the Body, Exits Tongue

Summana begins two thumb-widths above the navel and runs deep inside the chest, passing through the throat to exit at the tongue (fig. 2.4). There is no corresponding line on the back.

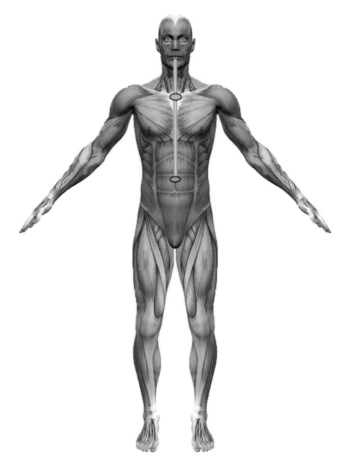

Fig. 2.4. The Summana line

Conditions: Asthma, bronchitis, chest pain, heart diseases, spasm of the diaphragm, nausea, cold, cough, throat problems, diseases of the digestive system, abdominal pain.

Sen 4: Kanlataree

Both Arms and Legs, Exits from the Ten Fingers and Toes

Kanlataree starts one thumb-width above the navel and separates into four branches (fig. 2.5). Two upper branches pass along the side of the ribcage through the inner scapulae to both arms,* moving downward to the wrists and exiting from all ten fingers. The two lower branches run downward on the medial sides of thighs and calves to the ankles, exiting from the ten toes.

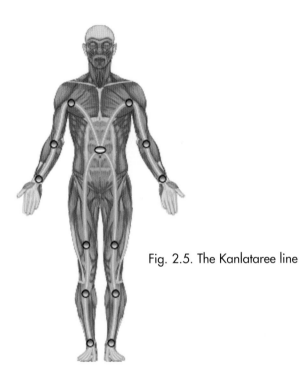

Fig. 2.5. The Kanlataree line

Conditions: Diseases of the digestive system, indigestion, hernia, paralysis of arms and legs, knee pain, jaundice, whooping cough, arthritis of the fingers, chest pain, shock, rheumatic heart disease and cardiac arrhythmia, sinusitis, pain in arms and legs, angina pectoris, epilepsy, schizophrenia, hysteria, various psychic diseases and mental disorders.

---

*Source: from the marble tablets at Wat Pho. Other sources describe different pathways for this line.

Sen 5: Hadsarangsri

Left Side of Body, Exits Left Eye

This Sen starts three thumb-widths from the navel on the left side of the abdomen (fig. 2.6). It runs down the medial side of the left thigh and leg to the left foot, passing along the base of all five toes. It then continues to the lateral side of the left foot moving upward along the lateral side of the left leg, close to the tibia. It continues up the left thigh and the left side of the ribcage, passing the left nipple and continuing upward to through the left side of the chin to exit at the left eye.

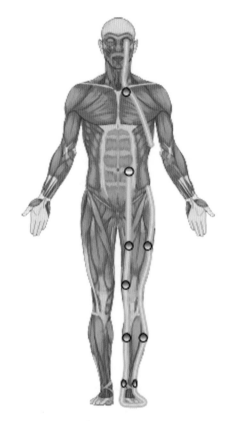

Fig. 2.6. The Hadsarangsri line

Conditions: Facial paralysis, toothache, throat ache, redness and swelling of the eye, fever, chest pain, mania, depressive psychosis, gastrointestinal diseases, diseases of the urogenital system, leg paralysis, arthritis of the knee joint, numbness of lower extremity, hernia.

Sen 6: Tawaree

Right Side of Body, Exits Right Eye

Tawaree runs the same pathway as Sen Hadsarangsri, on the other side of the body (fig. 2.7).

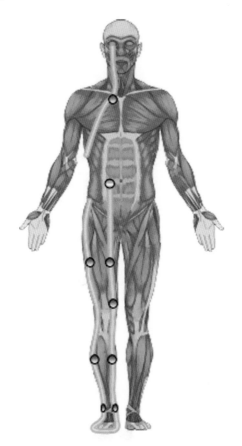

Fig. 2.7. The Tawaree line

Conditions: Same as Sen Hadsarangsri. Additional indications: jaundice and appendicitis.

Sen 7: Jantapusank

Left Side of Trunk, Exits Left Ear

This line starts four thumb-widths from the navel on the left side of the abdomen, and runs upward through the left breast to the left side of the neck, exiting at the left ear (fig. 2.8).

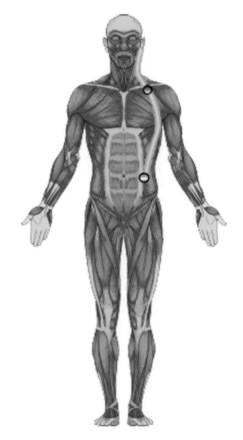

Fig. 2.8. The Jantapusank line

Conditions: Deafness, ear diseases, cough, facial paralysis, toothache, throat ache, chest pain, gastrointestinal diseases.

Sen 8: Rusum

Right Side of Trunk, Exits Right Ear

Rusum runs the same pathway as Sen Jantapusank, but on the right side of the body, exiting at the right ear (fig. 2.9).

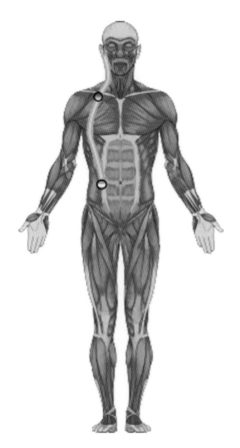

Fig. 2.9. The Rusum line

Conditions: Same as Sen Jantapusank: Deafness, ear diseases, cough, facial paralysis, toothache, throat ache, chest pain, gastrointestinal diseases.

Sen 9: Sukumang

Left Side of Abdomen, Exits Anus

Sukumang starts two thumb-widths under the navel and a little to the left, proceeding downward to exit at the anus (fig. 2.10). This Sen is generally treated with abdominal massage.

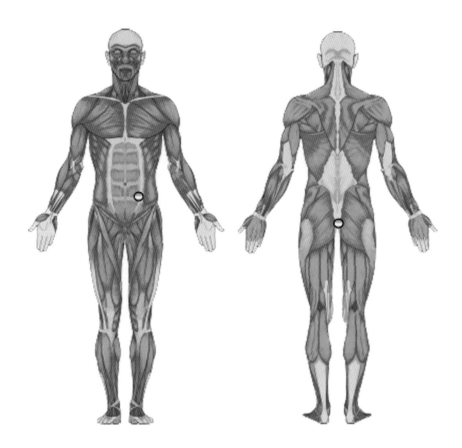

Fig. 2.10. The Sukumang line

Conditions: Hernia, frequent urination, female infertility, impotence, premature ejaculation, irregular menstruation, uterine bleeding, retention of urine, diarrhea, abdominal pain.

Sen 10: Sikinee

Right Side of Abdomen, Exits Sexual Organs and Urethra

This last Sen starts two thumb-widths under the navel and a little to the right (fig. 2.11). It runs downward to exit from the sex organs and the urethra. As with Sen Sukumung, therapy for Sen Sikinee is generally accomplished with abdominal massage.

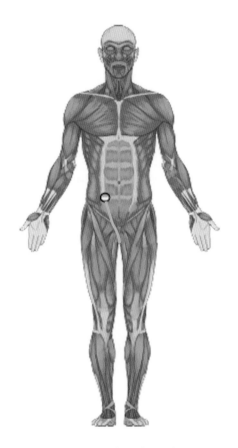

Fig. 2.11. The Sikinee line

Conditions: Same indications as for Sen Sukumang.

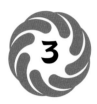

Chinese Medical Anatomy

The Tendinomuscular Meridians

The detailed meridian system of Chinese medicine extends well beyond the twelve organs and meridians that have now become familiar to many people in the West. In the practice of Chi Nei Ching, we focus our attention on the twelve tendinomuscular meridians—sometimes called the *sinew channels* or the *tendinomuscular regions*.

THE TENDINOMUSCULAR MERIDIANS

The tendinomuscular meridians are regions of muscle, tendon, and ligament that overlay the paths of the twelve regular meridians. Originating in the hands and feet, the twelve tendinomuscular regions ascend to the head and trunk. They are bilateral, appearing in mirror images on both sides of the body, and can have several branches. These regions are distributed deeply under the skin, connecting the bones and joints and maintaining the normal range of motion: their role is similar to the one ascribed to muscles in Western medicine.

Unlike the twelve primary meridans whose names they share, the tendinomuscular meridians do not run deep into the body to connect with the organs; rather, they remain at the surface, acting as an interface between the outside world and the regular meridians. They can affect the organs and body functions only indirectly, by virtue of their connection to the regular meridians. Knowledge of these tendinomuscular regions is used to guide traditional Thai therapeutic massage of the tendons (presented in chapter 5) and Tok Sen (described in detail in chapter 6).

The tendinomuscular meridians regulate the gross utilization of energy in the muscles. Massaging them regularly greatly increases the tone of the muscles, tendons, and fascia, and improves the range and efficiency of movement. Therapy along the tendinomuscular meridians is very effective in clearing blockages in muscles. It therefore improves circulation and helps reduce pain, soreness, and stiffness. Among the many areas of the body that can benefit from treatment of the tendinomuscular meridians are the neck and shoulders, where many people experience pain. In addition, because the traditional Thai massage is a holistic medicine, it recognizes that treating this region can actually help with ailments seemingly unrelated to the neck and shoulders.

Because the tendinomuscular regions connect to the primary meridians and indirectly to their organs, it is important to keep in mind that these muscle regions influence not just the muscles themselves but the functioning of internal organs as well. Thus a thorough knowledge of the muscle regions enables the therapist to treat assorted ailments; not just ones pertaining to the muscles and joints, but those pertaining to the organs also. Applying treatment to the correct region corresponding to a particular organ can help with maintenance or even health issues that relate to it.

Tendinomuscular Region of the Gall Bladder Meridian

The tendinomuscular region of the Gall Bladder meridian begins in the foot and ascends up the side of the leg. Detouring briefly to the buttocks area, the muscle region then runs up side of the trunk, neck, and head to end just below the ear (fig. 3.1).

Pathological symptoms include strained muscles of the lateral leg; an inability to bend the knee; muscle spasms or stiffness within the popliteal fossa; strain of the sacrum, pelvis, and lower ribs; pain in the chest; and an inability to turn the eyes to the left or right.

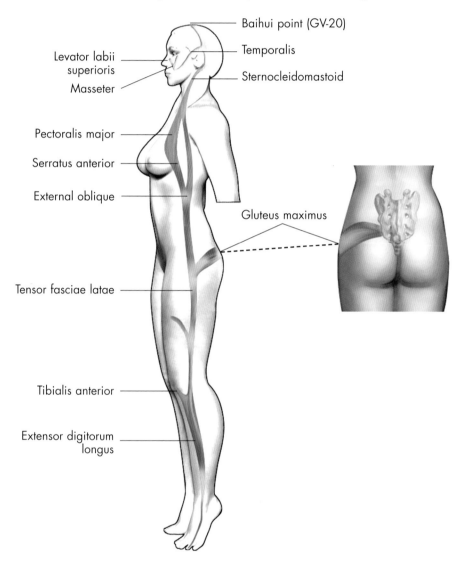

Baihui point (GV-20)

Levator labii superioris

Temporalis

Masseter

Sternocleidomastoid

Pectoralis major

Serratus anterior

External oblique

Gluteus maximus

Tensor fasciae latae

Tibialis anterior

Extensor digitorum longus

Fig. 3.1. Tendinomuscular region of the Gall Bladder meridian

Tendinomuscular Region of the Liver Meridian

The tendinomuscular region of the Liver meridian runs from the tip of the big toe along the inner portion of the leg, ending at the genital region (fig. 3.2). It is related not just to the ankle, knee, and thigh, but also to the reproductive organs.

Pathological symptoms include strained muscles of the big toe or top of the foot; pain in the anterior internal malleolus of the ankle; pain at the medial aspect of the knee and thigh; and dysfunction of the reproductive organs.

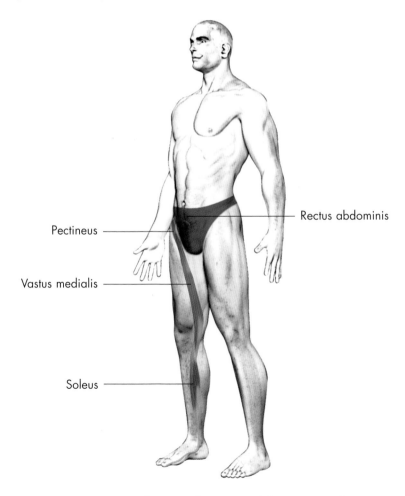

Pectineus

Vastus medialis

Soleus

Rectus abdominis

Fig. 3.2. Tendinomuscular region of the Liver meridian

Tendinomuscular Region of the Lung Meridian

The tendinomuscular region of the Lung meridian starts at the thumb and continues up the inner arm, into the chest area (fig. 3.3). In this case it is very close to the muscles of the lung itself. This muscle region influences the thumb and arm in addition to the respiratory system and lungs.

Pathological symptoms include strained, stiff, or spasming muscles of the thumb or arm. In more serious cases, there will be pain over the rib area, or a feeling of tightness in the chest.

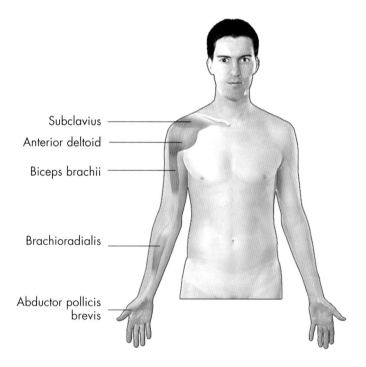

Subclavius
Anterior deltoid
Biceps brachii
Brachioradialis
Abductor pollicis brevis

Fig. 3.3. Tendinomuscular region of the Lung meridian

Tendinomuscular Region of the Large Intestine Meridian

The tendinomuscular region of the Large Intestine meridian runs from the index finger along the outer arm across the shoulder to the head (fig. 3.4). It reaches the side of the nose and crosses over the top of the head to the other side. A branch extends from the upper arm across the shoulder blade to the spine.

Pathological symptoms include strained muscles of the index finger or arm; stiffness, strained, or muscle spasms along the course of the large intestine channel; frozen shoulder; or an inability to rotate the neck from side to side.

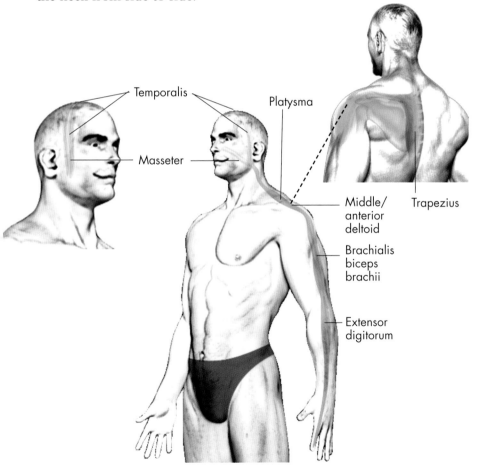

Fig. 3.4. Tendinomuscular region of the Large Intestine meridian

Tendinomuscular Region of the Stomach Meridian

The tendinomuscular region of the Stomach meridian begins in the foot and ascends up the front of the leg and trunk to the face (fig. 3.5). The areas of influence for this channel are rather substantial and include, but are not restricted to, the foot, lower leg and pelvis, stomach, breast area, and mouth. It also pertains to issues such as hernias, digestive issues, and jaw problems. This broad sphere of influence points out the profound and varying affects that the channels have as well as why they need to be correctly understood.

Pathological symptoms include strains or hardening of the muscles in the top of the foot; knotted or twisted muscles in the lower leg and thigh; swelling in the anterior pelvis region; hernia; spasms of the

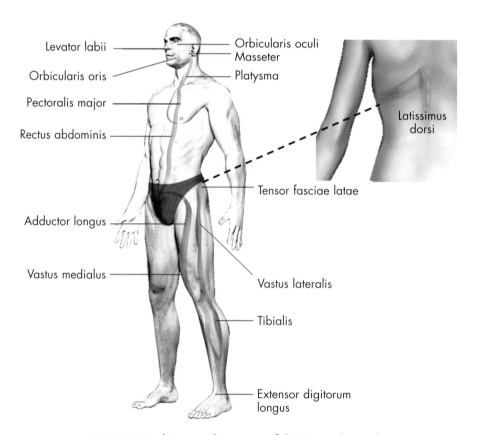

Fig 3.5. Tendinomuscular region of the Stomach meridian

abdominal muscles; spasms or stiffness of neck and cheek muscles; jaw problems; and eye spasms.

Tendinomuscular Region of the Spleen Meridian

The tendinomuscular region of the Spleen meridian starts at the big toe and continues up the inner aspect of the foot and leg to the genitals and the abdomen (fig. 3.6). A careful treatment of this tendinomuscular region is highly beneficial, allowing the practitioner to address problems from groin strains to chest issues.

Pathological symptoms include strained muscles of the big toe; pain in the internal malleolus of the ankle upon rotation; pain along the medial aspect of the knee and adductor muscles of the thigh; groin strain; and pain due to strained upper abdominal muscles and mid-thoracic vertebrae.

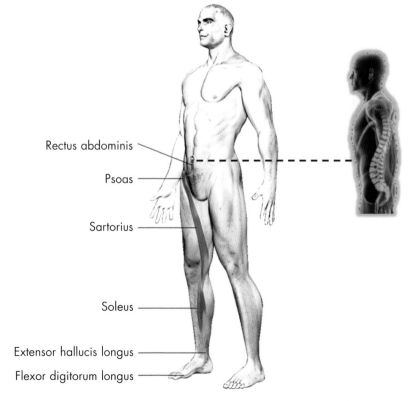

Rectus abdominis

Psoas

Sartorius

Soleus

Extensor hallucis longus

Flexor digitorum longus

Fig. 3.6. Tendinomuscular region of the Spleen meridian

Tendinomuscular Region of the Heart Meridian

The tendinomuscular region of the Heart meridian starts in the pinkie finger and runs up the inner arm to the chest (fig. 3.7). From the chest it runs town the midline to end at the navel. A practitioner can treat problems in this area including muscle spasms and difficulties along the Heart channel itself. It is obvious, as with the lungs, that this channel needs to be properly maintained because of the life-supporting nature of the heart.

Pathological symptoms include strained muscles of the little finger; stiff or strained muscles with spasm and/or pain along the course of the Heart channel, including internal cramping within the diaphragm and upper abdominal area.

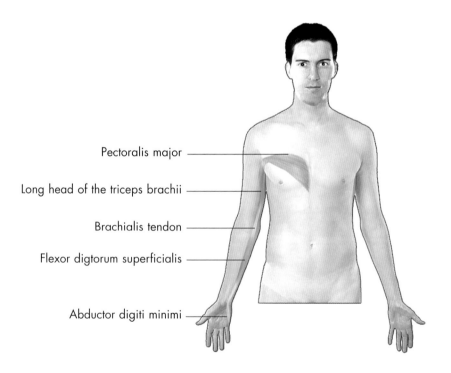

Pectoralis major

Long head of the triceps brachii

Brachialis tendon

Flexor digtorum superficialis

Abductor digiti minimi

Fig. 3.7. Tendinomuscular region of the Heart meridian

Tendinomuscular Region of the Small Intestine Meridian

The tendinomuscular region of the Small Intestine meridian begins at the tip of the pinkie finger and runs up the back of the arm to the scapula (fig. 3.8). From there is runs up the side of the neck and over the ear. Small branches spread out to reach the jawbone and the inner canthus of the eye. The range of this channel is vast and includes issues as varied as poor eyesight and elbow pain.

Pathological symptoms include strained muscles of the little finger or forearm; pain along the medial and posterior aspects of the elbow; pain in the posterior aspect of the axilla, neck, and scapula region; tinnitus related to earache; and poor vision.

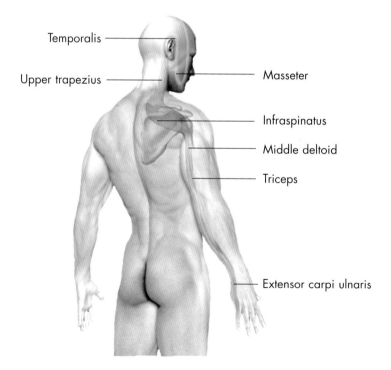

Fig. 3.8. Tendinomuscular region of the Small Intestine meridian

Tendinomuscular Region of the Urinary Bladder Meridian

The tendinomuscular region of the Urinary Bladder meridian has several branches that cover many regions of the body. It starts from the little toe, where several branches diverge and rise up the back of the leg through the buttocks and up the back (fig. 3.9). In the middle of the back, one branch extends around the scapula to the armpit, then rises across the chest into the neck and face. Another branch rises straight up to the occiput. Among the areas this channel influences are the neck and back. Proper treatment of this channel helps maintain the health of the back, shoulders, and bladder. Like all channels in the body, the Urinary Bladder muscle region needs regular maintenance to remain healthy.

Pathological symptoms include swelling and pain in the heels; stiffness or spasms along the backs of the legs; pain in the buttocks or

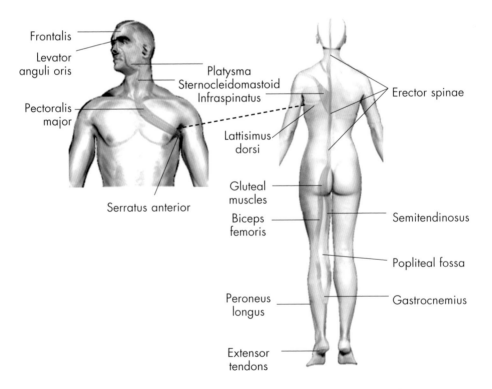

Fig. 3.9. Tendinomuscular region of the Urinary Bladder meridian

back; frozen shoulder; stiffness or spasms in the axillary and clavicle regions.

Tendinomuscular Region of the Kidney Meridian

The tendinomuscular region of the Kidney meridian begins in the little toe and runs along the sole of the foot to the inner ankle bone and up the inner aspect of the leg to the genitals (fig. 3.10). The influence of the Kidney channel is related to movement, and particularly to flexibility, as is required for bending and stretching.

Pathological symptoms include strained muscles on the bottom of the foot; pain or stiffness along the inside of the leg; back problems resulting in an inability to bend forward or backward, with difficulty in flexing or extending the head.

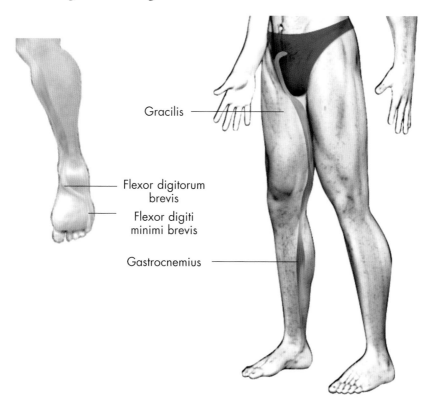

Gracilis

Flexor digitorum
brevis

Flexor digiti
minimi brevis

Gastrocnemius

Fig. 3.10. Tendinomuscular region of the Kidney meridian

Tendinomuscular Region of the Pericardium Meridian

The Pericardium meridian relates to the heart; specifically the membrane surrounding the heart. The tendinomuscular region of the Pericardium meridian begins at the tip of the middle finger, crosses the palm of the hand, and rises along in the middle of the inner arm to the axilla and the chest (fig. 3.11).

Pathological symptoms include strained muscles or tendons in the hands or wrist; spasms or pain along the inner aspect of the arm; chest pain and spasms.

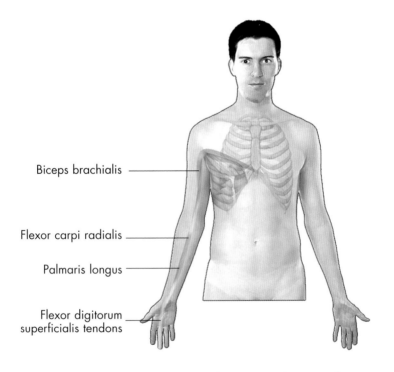

Biceps brachialis

Flexor carpi radialis

Palmaris longus

Flexor digitorum
superficialis tendons

Fig. 3.11. Tendinomuscular region of the Pericardium meridian

Tendinomuscular Region of the Triple Heater Meridian

The tendinomuscular region of the Triple Heater meridian runs from the tip of the fourth finger across the back of the hand and up the outside of the arm (fig. 3.12). It continues over the shoulder, up the neck, and along the side of the face. Its significance is in the treatment of extended muscles and involuntary muscle contractions in the neck and shoulders. The practitioner who knows this channel is able to facilitate the release of muscles that are hardened or stuck, providing movement that is more flexible and natural.

Pathological symptoms include strained muscles or tendons of the outer arm, shoulders, or neck.

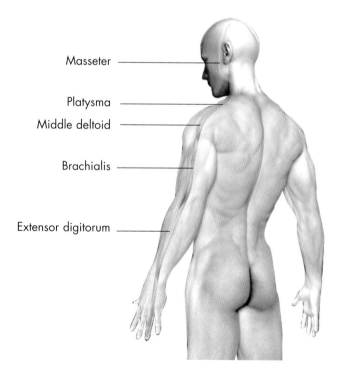

Masseter

Platysma

Middle deltoid

Brachialis

Extensor digitorum

Fig. 3.12. Tendinomuscular region of the Triple Heater meridian

PART 2

Treating the Muscles, Tendons, and Meridians with Chi Nei Ching

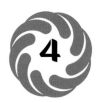

Preparing for Chi Nei Ching Practice

As a Chi Nei Ching practitioner or instructor, you have the responsibility of maintaining a clear, healthy body with a pure, strong flow of blood and chi. When you maintain yourself as the standard of healthy energy and a healthy body, you can then distinguish any problems or foreign elements that may be blocking your student's energy flow.

The task of cultivating and maintaining your energy can be broken down into three general categories: preparing yourself physically, emotionally, and energetically. These preparations are necessary to ensure that you can effectively interpret and guide your student's energies without getting overwhelmed. Below are some key practices for cultivating your energy in this way.

PREPARING YOURSELF PHYSICALLY
Maintaining a Strong and Healthy Body

When you are working to create the strong, healthy body necessary to practice Chi Nei Ching, bear in mind that energy flows to where it is needed. If your energy is lower than that of your students, their energy will flow to you and they will become weaker. We emphasize physical preparation because the tendons, muscles, fascia, channel systems, and bones draw in power that can be channeled to another person. The practices below will help you strengthen your physical body.

Iron Shirt Chi Kung

The Iron Shirt Chi Kung exercises allow you to draw energy from the earth, cosmos, and universe to strengthen the tendons and clean out and energize the fascia. This provides energetic protection and opens the channels so that they can receive more energy. With correct structural body alignment you can root yourself into the earth, creating an energetic grounding effect similar to the grounding wire of an electrical outlet. Proper grounding ensures that any excess energy you generate during your Chi Nei Ching practices will automatically release itself from your body and aura. By simply standing and packing in the Iron Shirt postures for five to ten minutes a day, you will root yourself to earth and build a strong body.

For details about the Iron Shirt practices, see Mantak Chia's *Iron Shirt Chi Kung.**

Tai Chi Chi Kung

By practicing Tai Chi you can learn to move your body as one unit using chi instead of muscle power. You can build inner strength by circulating energy through the channels, muscles, tendons, bones, and fascia. This ability is very important for energetic protection and for storing and channeling energy. The Universal Tao's Tai Chi Chi Kung, which can be learned very quickly, is a short but powerful way of achieving such results.

See *The Inner Structure of Tai Chi* for details about the basic Tai Chi Chi Kung form.†

---

*Mantak Chia, *Iron Shirt Chi Kung* (Rochester, Vt.: Destiny Books, 2006).
†Mantak Chia, *The Inner Structure of Tai Chi* (Rochester, Vt.: Destiny Books, 2005).

Bone Marrow Breathing

Bone Breathing uses the power of the mind, along with deep, relaxed inhalations, to establish an inward flow of external energy through the fingertips and toes. After external energy has been breathed into a particular area, muscle contractions are used to force the combined energies into the bones. By studying and practicing bone marrow breathing, you can cleanse and grow bone marrow, refresh the blood, and develop enormous power. You can develop the ability to channel energy through breathing while using less muscular force and passing on more energy.

For detailed instructions on Bone Marrow Breathing practices, see Mantak Chia's *Bone Marrow Nei Kung.**

The Five-Element Diet

The five-element style of cooking that pervades much of the world of Chinese cuisine is featured in many wonderful restaurants. In fact, the practices of this type of cooking are a part of every Asian culture. Asian cooks balance their food in five ways, categorizing foods according to five tastes, five colors, hot, cold, and pH balance. Then the foods are combined and beautifully prepared.

The stomach, spleen, and saliva sort the food and distribute it to the organs according to taste and color. Each color and taste feeds energy to a particular organ group. Each organ will accept only that energy designed for it by nature.

A balanced diet is one that provides each organ with its own kind of energy. Each organ's energy then feeds primary energy to certain systems in the body. To nourish the body's various systems, you have to plan your meals accordingly. Thus, a balanced diet has equal parts of the following five tastes and colors:

---

*Mantak Chia, *Bone Marrow Nei Kung* (Rochester, Vt.: Destiny Books, 2006).

- The liver and gallbladder like food that is green and sour. This food feeds the nerves.
- The heart and small intestine like food that is bitter and red. This food feeds the heart and its vessels.
- The spleen, pancreas, and stomach like food that is sweet. This food feeds the muscles. This does not mean adding sugar or sweeteners but refers to food that is naturally sweet.
- The lungs and large intestine like food that is spicy and light colored. This food feeds the skin.
- The kidneys and bladder like food that is dark and salty. This food feeds the bones. This does not mean adding salt but refers to food that is naturally salty.

Food also has cold/hot and yin/yang properties that are important to understand and balance. Many macrobiotic diets are incomplete because they balance food only according to yin and yang and do not employ the five phases of energy theory.

For more on the five-element diet, see our book *Cosmic Nutrition.**

PREPARING YOURSELF EMOTIONALLY
The Fusion Practices

In addition to a strong, healthy body, you need to work from a clear emotional base to practice Chi Nei Ching. You cannot help anyone if you are full of negative emotional energy. The Fusion of the Five Elements practices, described in Mantak Chia's *Fusion of the Five Elements*, will allow you to clear out your negative emotional energy and transform it into positive emotional energy.[†] These are very powerful and effective meditations and formulations for balancing the emotions.

When you practice Fusion of the Five Elements, you will learn

---

*Mantak Chia and William U. Wei, *Cosmic Nutrition* (Rochester, Vt.: Destiny Books, 2012).
[†]Mantak Chia, *Fusion of the Five Elements* (Rochester, Vt.: Destiny Books, 2007).

how the five energy phases and their related organs can interact with one another. This technique teaches you how to construct an internal system of turbines, transformers, and vortexes that can be used to cleanse the emotions. If you know how to engage this system, you can switch it on while you are massaging someone and any negative and sick energies trying to invade your body can be quickly neutralized.

PREPARING YOURSELF ENERGETICALLY
Connecting with Your Sources of Energy

The first step in preparing your energy for Chi Nei Ching practices is to establish a strong connection with the sources of that energy: the universal, human plane, and earth energies. As you connect with these forces, you can unify and blend them into one energy. You will be strong and the energy flowing through you will be of the correct quality and quantity to help your student.

Open as Many Channels as Possible

The more channels you open, the better off you are. To receive energy, it is important to open at least the two major channels of the Microcosmic Orbit—the Functional Channel and Governor Channel (see pages 54–55 at the end of this chapter to find directions for the Microcosmic Orbit meditation). It is better still to add the Thrusting and Belt Channels as described in *Cosmic Fusion*.* By doing so you will know firsthand the way your energy flows. Then you can direct and draw in healthy energy and use it to burn sick energy out of your system. By first opening the energy channels within yourself, you become more efficient as a healer and can avoid succumbing to the illnesses that you are removing from another.

---

*Meditations for opening the Thrusting and Belt Channels can be found in *Cosmic Fusion* (Rochester, Vt.: Destiny Books, 2007), 145–97.

Practice Meditation Daily and After Each Session

To maintain your energy, meditate every day to reconnect with the outer forces and burn out sick and undesired energy. Often, those who lose touch with these outer forces find their egos rising and expanding. In such a situation you may believe you have the power to heal others, but really you are not equipped and can easily pick up sick energy.

Ideally, you would practice the Inner Smile, Microcosmic Orbit, and Healing Hands meditations each day. These meditations can be found at the end of this chapter, on pages 53–57. After each session, you can practice meditations to clear your energy.

Protect Yourself from Surface Sick Energy

When helping someone it is possible to accumulate sick energy on the surface of the skin of your hands and arms. Do not allow it to go beyond the shoulders and enter the body. If you practice daily, your mind's power can hold back the encroachment of the sick energy.

There are many different theories on how to get rid of this unwanted surface energy. Some people advocate washing the hands. If you do this, make sure that you use cold, running water, or else you can drive the energy further into your body.

Another method is to place your hands on a surface conductive to earth energy and connected to a ground (e.g., a water pipe). Iron will do, as will a brick or cement wall that has a footing. The conductive material will pass the sick energy down to the ground, which can help neutralize it. With some sick energies this grounding method is not effective or powerful enough. Therefore, our advice is that you meditate as well so that you are sure to be clean. Be sure that you are free of sick energy before ending your meditation. You may feel coldness in the hands, itchy skin, and a lack of energy. Meditate until you feel warmth in your hands; it will burn out the sick energy.

Trees, especially pines, are excellent for taking sick energy into the earth, as are other outdoor plants. Potted plants, though, can absorb only limited amounts of sick energy, as they are not directly connected to the earth.

HEALING WITH LOVE FROM THE HEART'S CENTER

When people come to you for healing, you should wish them well with all your heart. Give them your love, kindness, and openness, and you will feel your heart open. The healing force from the universe will pour down to you and out to the people simultaneously. Learning Iron Shirt Chi Kung is very important because it is the practice that will allow you to ground yourself when working with a student. This will help you ground your energy and help send the student's sick energy into the ground. You will also learn to feel the kindness, gentleness, and openness of the earth force and will pass the earth force into your student.

Giving the gift of healing energy keeps the heart channels open, and both the practitioner and student benefit. Practice the Microcosmic Orbit circulation; concentrate on the point opposite the heart and feel it connect to the heart center in the front. This will help open the heart. Feel the back and the front connected like a funnel. Once the heart is open, it will be very easy to receive energy from the universe. Opening the Microcosmic Orbit is very important, since this will allow the energy to circulate, balance, recycle, and transform. The meditative practices of the Universal Tao will enable you to connect with the heavenly force from above and the earth force from below. Combine them into a powerful healing force—a healing force that can be used to heal yourself and others.

MEDITATIONS FOR DAILY PRACTICE

 ## The Inner Smile

1. Be aware of smiling cosmic energy in front of you and breathe it into your eyes.

2. Allow smiling energy to enter the point between your eyebrows. Let it flow into your nose and cheeks, and let it lift up the corners of your mouth, bringing your tongue to rest on your palate.

3. Smile down to your neck, throat, thyroid, parathyroid, and thymus.

4. Smile into your heart, feeling joy and love spread out from there to the lungs, liver, spleen, pancreas, kidneys, and genitals.

5. Bring smiling energy into the eyes, then down to the mouth.

6. Swallow saliva as you smile down to your stomach, small intestine (duodenum, jejunum, and ileum), large intestine (ascending colon, transverse colon, and descending colon), rectum, and anus.

7. Smile, and look upward about 3 inches into your mid-eyebrow point and pituitary gland.

8. Direct your smile to the Third Room, the small cavity deep in the center of your brain. Feel the room expand and grow with the bright golden light shining through the brain.

9. Smile into the thalamus, pineal gland (Crystal Room), and the left and right sides of the brain.

10. Smile to the midbrain and the brain stem, then to the base of your skull.

11. Smile down to the seven cervical vertebrae, the twelve thoracic vertebrae, the five lumbar vertebrae, then the sacrum and the tailbone.

12. Refresh the loving, soothing smile energy in your eyes, then smile down the front, middle, and back lines in succession. Now do all of them at once, feeling bathed in a cooling waterfall or glowing sunshine of cosmic energy, smiles, joy, and love.

13. Gather all the smiling energy in your navel area—about 1.5 inches

inside your body. Spiral that energy with your mind or your hands from the center point to the outside. (Don't go above the diaphragm or below the pubic bone.)

14. Men spiral clockwise 36 times, then counterclockwise 24 times, returning energy toward the center. Women spiral out counterclockwise 36 times, then inward clockwise 24 times. Finish by storing energy safely in the navel.

Opening the Microcosmic Orbit

Sit comfortably on the sitz bones, with your back straight and chin tucked in slightly. The nine points of the feet should be on the floor, with the shoulders relaxed and the scapulae rounded.

1. Place your right hand on the navel center and the left hand on the pubic bone/sexual center. Send energy from the right hand to the left, then spiral energy at the sexual center with your mind and eyes: 36 times counterclockwise, then 36 times clockwise. Inhale and exhale into the sexual center 9–18 times, feeling chi accumulate.

2. Move your left hand to the perineum, feeling energy radiate down from the navel and sexual center. Spiral energy with mind/eye power at the perineum 36 times counterclockwise then 36 times clockwise, then inhale and exhale into the perineum 9–18 times.

3. Gather energy into a chi ball at the lower tan tien and rotate it top to front to bottom to back; then bring the chi ball into the perineum.

4. Place your left hand on your sacrum and coccyx, right hand on the sexual center. Pull up lightly on the perineum and anus, drawing energy up from the right hand to the left. Spiral this energy at the sacrum and coccyx 36 times in each direction, then inhale and exhale into the area 3–9 times.

5. Move your left hand to the Door of Life and let chi radiate to that point. Spiral a chi ball there 36 times in each direction, then inhale and exhale into the Door of Life 9–18 times.

6. Place your right hand on your sacrum and use your left hand to add the following points to the orbit: T11, the wing point between T5 and T6 (opposite the heart), then the C7 point, Jade Pillow, back of the crown, and top of the crown, and the mid-eyebrow point. Spiral a chi ball at each point 36 times in each direction, then inhale and exhale into the point 3–9 times.

7. Press the tip of your tongue against your palate then release it, repeating 9–18 times. Knock your teeth together 18–36 times, then lightly clench and release them. Rotate a chi ball at the palate 36 times each way, then inhale and exhale into the palate 3–9 times.

8. Use your left hand to add the throat center, heart center, and solar plexus center: collect energy at each point and spiral it 36 times in each direction, then inhale and exhale into the point.

9. Return energy to the navel and spiral it 36 times in each direction. Inhale and exhale into the navel point 3–9 times, feeling energy pulsing behind the navel.

10. Continue to guide the energy flow through the Microcosmic Orbit as many times as you like, then relax and let the energy flow however it wants to. Spend 5–10 minutes at this stage, just feeling your body dissolve into your Original Chi, resting in a state of emptiness.

11. Collect all the energy at your navel and in front of the kidneys. Spiral the energy around the navel 36 times outward and 24 times inward. Men rotate clockwise outward and counterclockwise inward, women the opposite.

The Healing Hands Meditation

When you place your hands on a client, you are opening a circuit that can communicate a great deal of information in both directions. To be sure that you are giving and receiving this information correctly, it is important to develop the energy in your hands and fingers. The Healing Hands meditation will develop sensitivity, and help you to feel the energy in your student and yourself. This practice increases the ability of your hands to channel the universal, human plane (cosmic particle), and earth energies. You will be able to feel the energy emerging from your palms and fingers as you touch your student.

⟳ Part 1: Meditating to Expand the Aura

1. Practice the Inner Smile meditation; then bring energy to your navel center. Practice the Fusion meditations, forming four pakuas and transforming negative emotions into positive healing forces. Then form a pearl.
2. Circulate the pearl in your Microcosmic Orbit faster and faster until it expands outward from your body, filling your aura with a warm sensation. Absorb violet and red lights from the North Star and the Big Dipper above you; absorb golden light from the cosmic particle energy; absorb blue light from the earth into your navel.
3. When your aura has expanded, maintain a distance of at least 2 feet from other people.

⟳ Part 2: Channeling Force through the Palms

1. Hold both hands in front of your eyes and use the corners of both eyes to gaze at the palms' centers. Use your mind and eyes to absorb cosmic chi into your right palm, then send the chi from your right palm and fingers into your left palm and fingers. Repeat 9 times.
2. Hold your hands facing each other but not touching, and feel the energy travel between them. Gradually spread your hands apart while maintaining the chi connection between them. Pull them together and apart 9–18 times.

⊚ Parts 3 and 4: Growing the Auras of Your Fingers

1. With both palms facing your eyes, gaze from the corners of the right eye at the right hand's fingers. Focus on the tip of the index finger and its aura. Using the energy of your eyes, expand the aura of this fingertip, making the energy cool and pleasant. Then grow the auras of your other fingers in turn: middle finger, thumb, ring finger, and pinkie.

2. Inhale energy into your left hand and fingers, and gaze at the tip of your thumb. Grow the thumb's aura, then turn your gaze to each of the other fingers, growing the index finger, middle finger, ring finger, and pinkie finger's auras.

3. Place your hands on your knees with your palms facing upward. On your left hand, form a circle with your thumb and index finger, keeping the other fingers straight. On your right hand, form a circle with your thumb and the ring and pinkie fingers, keeping the index and middle fingers straight.

4. Keeping your fingers in these circles, use your mind and eyes to absorb cosmic particle force through the fingers of the left hand. Send it up the outside of the left arm and shoulder to the back of the left ear and across the crown. Blend this energy with the universal force entering through the crown, then send this combined energy down to the right ear, right shoulder, the outside of the right arm and hand, and then the index and middle fingers. Send this energy out through these fingers and receive it again through the extended fingers of the left hand. Repeat for 18 or 36 cycles.

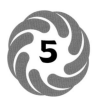

Nuad Thai
Thai Therapeutic Massage

Thai massage, or Nuad Thai, is an ancient technique that provides many benefits, including increased energy, stress relief, improved physical and emotional balance, improved circulation, detoxification of the body, and an increased sense of well-being. This corrective has met the test of time and is a technique that is especially useful in the modern age of hard work, tension, and stress, which cause a wide variety of maladies throughout the body, mind, and spirit. Long considered a sacred art and associated with Thai Buddhist practice, Nuad Thai has been handed down for centuries. To this day, it is associated with Buddhism and Buddhist temples throughout the country.

THE BENEFITS OF THAI MASSAGE

Nuad Thai improves health and well-being in direct and also indirect ways. Initially, it improves circulation, thereby strengthening the heart and the circulatory system. By increasing circulation and also removing blockages in the muscles and tendons, Thai massage helps the tendinomuscular system to regain its elasticity, which brings about improved mobility and energy. Thus, for example, exercise is easier and the muscles become stronger. The tendons also become more flexible and this helps prevent injury.

Thai massage therapy also helps to improve digestion. This is partly because the entire digestive tract is restored to, or maintained at, an optimal level of elasticity. Even relatively simple issues, such as minor indigestion, can be relieved with the appropriate therapy.

A more long-term result of Thai massage is the way it softens armored areas of the body. Consequently, healing channels in the body are opened and toxic material dissipates. This is useful not just for short-term healing but for removing entrenched stagnation and blockages. Because of the holistic nature of our systems, this can have far-reaching positive consequences such as the reduction of swelling in different parts of the body.

Perhaps the greatest benefit of Thai massage, however, is its ability to reduce pain from a multitude of causes. One way to understand pain is to see it as a vibration coming from an external source that has been locked into the tendon. The vibration pulls on the muscle, creating aches and pains. Frequently, these aches and pains spread through the entire length of the tendinomuscular meridian. It is similar to when a person exercises vigorously or engages in a strenuous workout, and the next day their muscles are stiff from a buildup of lactic acid. Most of us know that this stiffness has to be "worked out" so that the built-up acid dissipates. It is also possible, however, to dissipate these aches and pains with the correct use of massage.

HAND TECHNIQUES FOR THAI MASSAGE

The hand techniques of Chi Nei Tsang are used to massage most surfaces of the body, including the abdomen, arteries, muscles, tendons, spine, shoulder blades, coccyx, arms, legs, feet, joints, hands, neck, and meridian lines. The most common hand techniques are the finger press, spiraling, hand scooping, and shaking techniques. Each of these can be performed with either one or both hands.

By massaging the skin and stimulating its surface, you can draw

the pressure and toxicity from deep within the tendons and muscles—
and indeed from all parts of the body—to the surface.

Finger Press

Using the tip of your thumb, forefinger, or middle finger, press gently
into the point. If your student feels comfortable with this gentle pressure, you can begin to press a little bit more deeply.

Spiral

Massage the point in small, tight, clockwise circular motions, loosening the skin and the tissue underneath it. To cover large areas, work
outward in a spiral extending from the center of the point into the
surrounding muscle.

If you are using both hands, gently press a point with the thumbs
or forefingers together.

Scoop

With your fingers together, press the side of your hand into the tissue
and "scoop" it downward or outward.

Shake

Use either your index or your middle finger to press on the knot or
problem area. Move your finger quickly up and down or from side to
side. Use two or three fingers to cover a larger area.*

---

*For more detailed information about these and other Chi Nei Tsang techniques, see
Mantak Chia's *Chi Nei Tsang* (Rochester, Vt.: Destiny Books, 2007), 162–68.

HOW TO PERFORM A THAI MASSAGE

Thai massage can be done as a full-body massage or used to address problem areas only. For each area of the body being treated, the practitioner first evaluates the conditions of the muscles and tendons by looking at and palpating the muscles, tendons, and joints. When areas of tension or armoring are identified, the practitioner can then apply one or more of the hand techniques described above to release that tension.

 ## Opening Stretch

Before beginning the massage, it is a good idea to relax the whole body and stretch the tendons as follows.

1. With the student lying on her back, the practitioner stands or sits at the feet and takes the student's heels in hand.
2. Rock the legs gently from side to side a few times.
3. Raise the legs a few inches and rock them again from side to side.
4. Place your thumbs and palm-heels—or the ulnar edge of your hand—against the base of your student's toes. Have her press her toes against your hands as you apply a little bit of resistance; this simple stretch can activate all the tendons of the body.
5. Take your student's heels once more and rock the legs gently from side to side. Slowly release the heels to the table.

Head and Neck

The neck's many layered muscles are required for supporting and turning the relatively heavy head (see fig. 5.1 on page 62). For many people, the head and neck are centers of frequent tension and pain. Eye strain, grinding or clenching teeth, lymphatic overload, and sinus issues can all cause chronic head and neck pain. Accident or trauma can also cause problems in this region. Massage of the head and neck can be enormously helpful in relieving neck and head pain from any source.

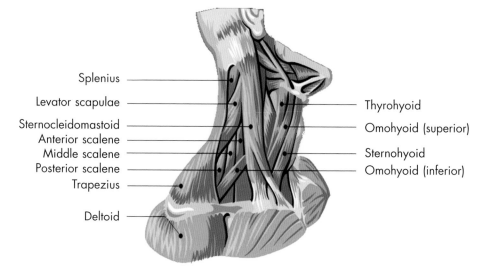

Splenius

Levator scapulae

Sternocleidomastoid

Anterior scalene

Middle scalene

Posterior scalene

Trapezius

Deltoid

Thyrohyoid

Omohyoid (superior)

Sternohyoid

Omohyoid (inferior)

Fig. 5.1. Lateral neck muscles

 ## Massaging the Head and Neck

Most of the Sen lines, as well as the tendinomuscular regions of the gallbladder, stomach, large intestine, small intestine, bladder, and Triple Heater channels, run through the neck, as shown in chapters 2 and 3. It is helpful to be aware of these meridians as you work.

1. Ask the student to turn his head slowly toward the right shoulder. At the same time, gently palpate the exposed left side of the neck to feel for areas of tension and/or armoring. If necessary, you can apply a little resistance to the side of the face to make the muscles and tendons more obvious.

2. Repeat this step on the right side of the neck as the student turns his head toward the left.

3. Have the student tip his head slowly forward and backward, again applying resistance if necessary. Look for areas of tension along the sides and back of the neck.

4. Use the finger techniques of Chi Nei Tsang to release the tight and armored areas of the neck. Be sure to massage the whole region from the jaw bone to the collarbone.

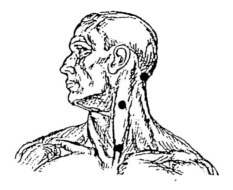

Fig. 5.2. Points on the neck

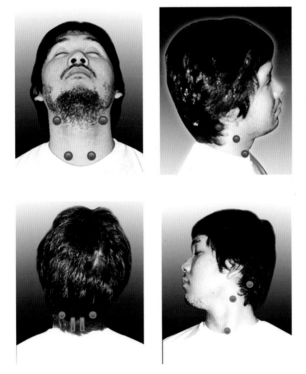

Fig. 5.3. Anterior and lateral vertebral muscles in the neck

Some of the significant points in the region are highlighted in figures 5.2 and 5.3. In addition, figure 5.1 shows the different muscles in the area of the neck.

Shoulder and Upper Arm

Many people suffer from shoulder and neck pain due to muscle pain, tension, or injury of some sort. Even routines such as using a computer for long periods of time or poor posture can result in pain in the shoulder area. This type of pain can negatively impact the quality of a person's life; the good news is that the appropriate therapy is frequently able to relieve this chronic pain.

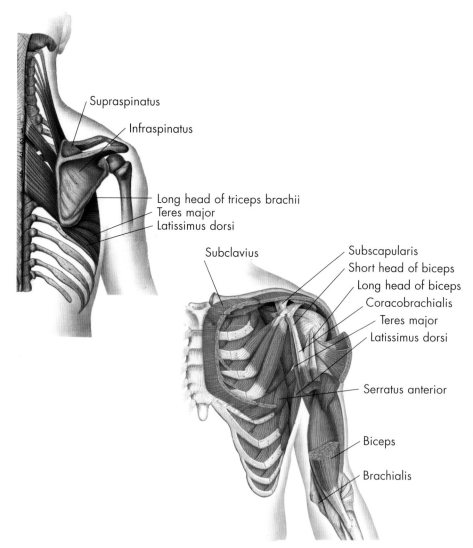

Fig. 5.4. Muscles of the shoulder and connecting regions

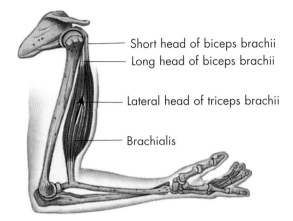

Short head of biceps brachii
Long head of biceps brachii

Lateral head of triceps brachii

Brachialis

Fig. 5.5. The biceps muscle and tendons

What is experienced as shoulder pain can actually originate in other areas of the body; the spine, for example. Figure 5.6 shows the relationship of the shoulders to other nearby areas.

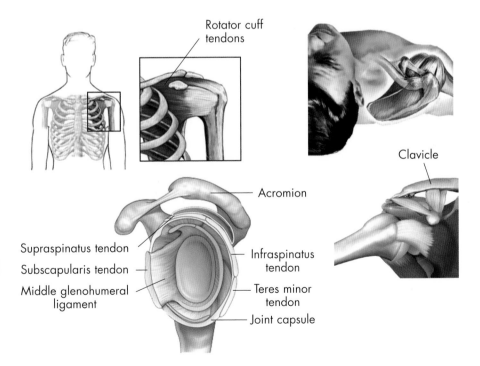

Rotator cuff tendons

Clavicle

Acromion

Supraspinatus tendon
Subscapularis tendon
Middle glenohumeral ligament

Infraspinatus tendon
Teres minor tendon
Joint capsule

Fig. 5.6. The shoulder's relationship to the neck and arm

Evaluating and Treating the Shoulders

1. While the student is seated, stand at her left side and place your left hand on the front of her left shoulder. Your fingertips should be pressing into the muscles and tendons on the trunk, just below the outer edge of the clavicle (fig. 5.7).

2. With your right hand, raise the student's arm to chest height, then stretch it slowly outward and toward the back. At the same time, your left hand should be holding the tendon under the shoulder at approximately the chest region. Essentially, the tendon needs to be activated by stretching and then be pressed.

3. Next bring the student's arm forward, stretching it across the chest as you palpate the tendons and muscles of the shoulder. Again stretch and press against the tendon to bring chi and blood to it.

4. Stretch the student's arm forward and gently twist the wrist in both directions to stretch the tendons.

5. Massage the tendinomuscular regions of the lung and large intestine meridians, and the small intestine and Triple Heater meridians as shown in chapter 3, using standard Chi Nei Tsang strokes.

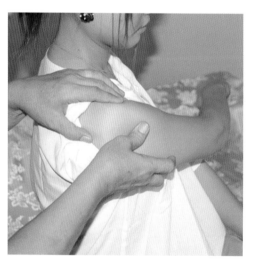 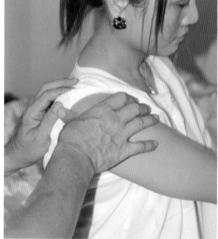

Fig. 5.7. Massaging the shoulder

6. Massage thoroughly all around the scapula, paying special attention to the inner and upper borders, which can collect a lot of tension (fig 5.8).

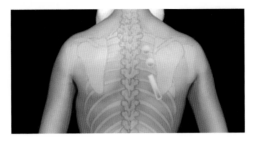

Fig. 5.8. Massage points on the inner scapula

The Upper Body and Anger

Anger can influence many parts of the body. While anger is a natural human emotion, if it is channeled incorrectly problems can result. That includes not only personal or interpersonal problems but problems that influence the body. Think of the posture of a person who is extremely angry and it is evident that the entire position of their body changes, including the shoulder region. Such anger has the possibility of causing stress and ultimately pain in the shoulder or other areas that have locked this stress or negativity inside. Chronic or habitual anger has the potential to change the center of gravity of the body, even moving it up into the area of the throat, chest, or shoulders.

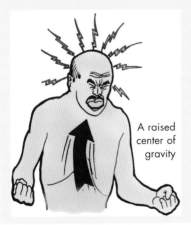

A raised center of gravity

The proper massage therapy can greatly assist with not only relieving stress, but in managing anger, depression, and anxiety as well.

Fig. 5.9. Excessive anger can bring the center of gravity high up in the chest or the throat.

Elbow and Lower Arm

Numerous tendon lines—and tendinomuscular meridians—run the length of the arm from the shoulder to the hand (fig. 5.10). These tendons are prone to injuries and repetitive strain disorders like tennis elbow and carpal tunnel syndrome. In addition, the many joints of the hands and wrists are vulnerable to arthritis and other inflammatory conditions, many of which respond very well to Thai massage techniques.

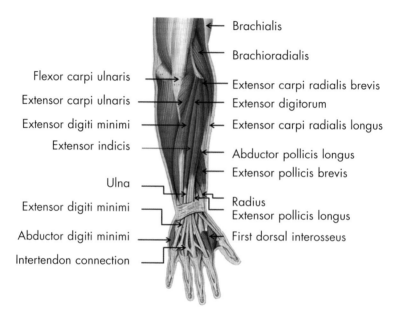

Brachialis

Brachioradialis

Flexor carpi ulnaris

Extensor carpi radialis brevis

Extensor carpi ulnaris

Extensor digitorum

Extensor digiti minimi

Extensor carpi radialis longus

Extensor indicis

Abductor pollicis longus

Extensor pollicis brevis

Ulna

Radius
Extensor pollicis longus

Extensor digiti minimi

Abductor digiti minimi

First dorsal interosseus

Intertendon connection

Fig. 5.10. Muscles and tendons of the arm

 Evaluating and Treating the Arms and Elbows

After massaging the length of the arm it is helpful to focus on the elbow, where many muscles, tendons, and nerves can get strained and tangled. Thorough massage in this area helps release blockages in the tendons, nerves, and muscles, and it also helps the muscles become more naturally elastic.

1. Extend the arm slightly outward and twist it gently from the wrist. At the same time, palpate the tendons around the elbow to feel for tight and constricted areas.
2. Gently massage down the arm from the shoulder to the hand, changing or repeating strokes as necessary (fig. 5.11).

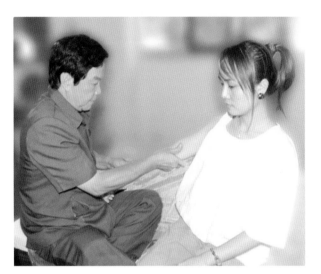
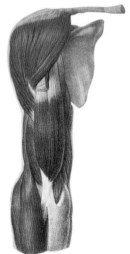

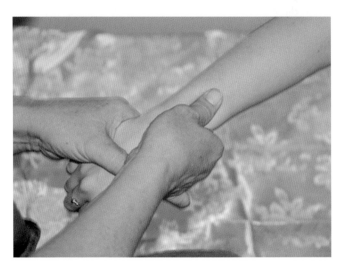

Fig. 5.11. Massaging the arm and elbow

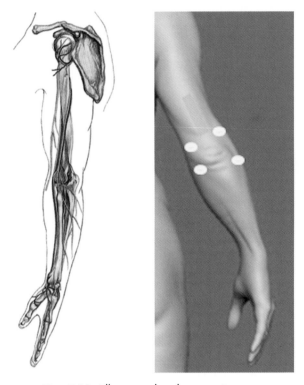

Fig. 5.12. Elbow tendon therapeutic massage

3. Massage the points around the elbow tendons as shown in fig. 5.12. Do not press directly on the elbow bone itself, but apply pressure to a single point while sliding outward. Then move on to the next point.
4. Repeat steps 1–3 until the elbow and arm feel clear and unconstrained.

Wrists and Hands

Pain in the wrist, particularly down into the thumb, can be quite debilitating. One reason for this is that lots of chi resides there.

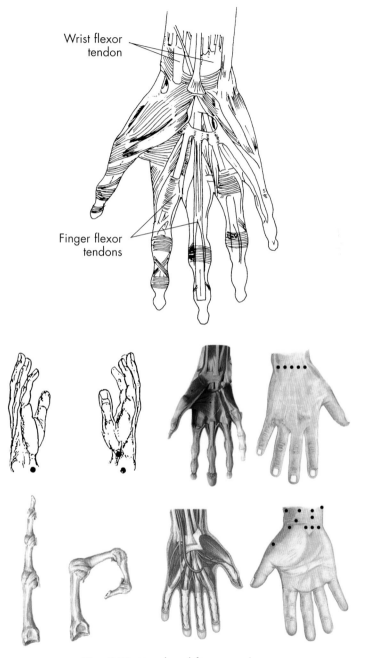

Fig. 5.13. Hand and finger tendons

Evaluating and Treating the Wrists and Hands

1. Gently move the wrist up and down while palpating the tendons on the front and back sides (fig. 5.14).
2. Massage any areas of tension or pain.
3. Next, gently twist the thumb back and forth as you palpate and massage the tendons that run through it. Often, the area of the thumb that has an issue is on the palm of the hand down toward the wrist. The bone can be felt there as well as the associated tendons.
4. Gently rotate each finger in turn, palpating and massaging the tendons associated with it. Twist, then release, twist and release, repeating until the tendons are looser. There is a delicacy about the fingers in particular and care must be taken. Of course patience is necessary too.

Hand Reflexology

It is interesting to note that reflexology systems connect different regions of the hand to various other parts of the body—for example, to the head, brain, legs, and feet, as well as many other areas. There is a kinship here to the philosophy behind acupuncture.

Even without learning the specific correspondences for each area of the hand, you can massage it carefully to treat other bodily ailments. Find the tendon area alongside the bone first, then proceed to work areas along it with pressure and movement away from the bone. The technique is to search for areas that are painful and then to work them out. A stomachache, headache, or even toothache can be treated this way. As with all therapy, caution is in order with some situations. For example, if an individual is pregnant the practitioner should not work her hand in this manner.

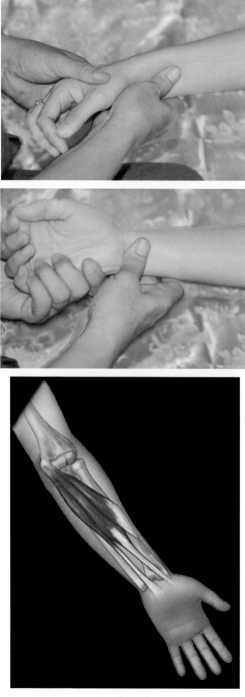

Fig. 5.14. Hand tendon massage

Spine

The spinal column is of major importance in the function and well-being of the human body, influencing and facilitating a myriad of significant functions related to motion, sensation, and organ function. In order to accomplish these tasks, the nerves within the spinal cord must be protected, and there must be appropriate alignment and cushioning of the spinal vertebrae.

However, these vertebrae are rather easily displaced, which can cause a variety of problems including pain, numbness, and dysfunction of the organs or limbs. If nerves are pinched or compressed between two vertebrae, the pain and debility can be quite severe. Vertebral displacement can be caused by injury, chronic strain, fatigue, muscle spasms, aging, or other factors. Fortunately, many of these issues can be successfully treated with skilled massage therapy.

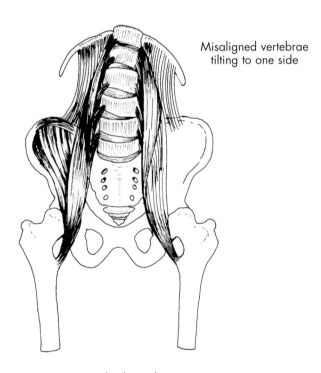

Misaligned vertebrae
tilting to one side

Fig. 5.15. Vertebral misalignment can
cause a variety of problems.

The misalignment shown in figure 5.15—caused by a short psoas muscle on one side—can create further misalignments throughout the spine (fig. 5.16).

As shown in the table on page 77, the extraordinary number of issues that can result from misalignment range from insomnia and headache to allergies and skin issues; from deafness to speaking problems and breathing to coronary issues.

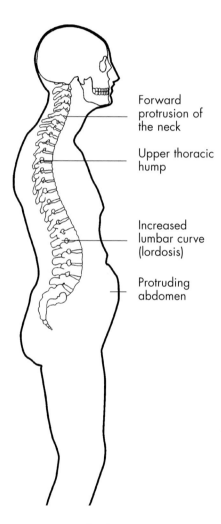

Forward protrusion of the neck

Upper thoracic hump

Increased lumbar curve (lordosis)

Protruding abdomen

Fig. 5.16. Swayback misalignment caused by a shortened psoas

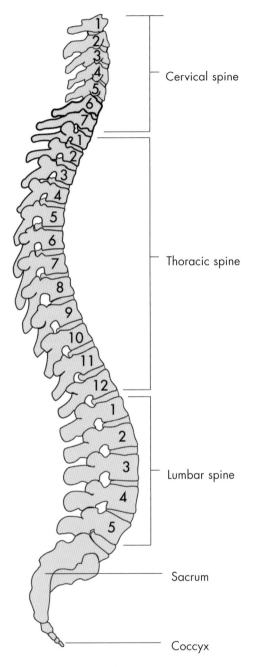

Cervical spine

Thoracic spine

Lumbar spine

Sacrum

Coccyx

Fig. 5.17. The spine

CORRESPONDENCES OF VERTEBRAL SEGMENTS
TO OTHER PARTS OF THE BODY

VERTEBRA	ORGAN FIELD	CONSEQUENCES OF DISPLACEMENT OR DYSFUNCTION
1 Cervical	Blood supply to the brain and inner/middle ear	Headache, insomnia, pituitary disease, high blood pressure, tiredness, dizziness
2 Cervical	Eyes, auditory nerve, tongue	Allergy, eye and ear symptoms
3 Cervical	Outer ear, teeth, trigeminal nerve	Trigeminal neuralgia, acne
4 Cervical	Nose, lips, mouth	Deafness, polyps
5 Cervical	Vocal cords	Hoarseness, vocal cord inflammation
6 Cervical	Neck, shoulders, tonsils	Pain in the neck and upper arm
7 Cervical	Thyroid gland, shoulder joint, elbow	Thyroid problems, tennis elbow
1 Thoracic	Forearms, hands, esophagus	Cough, breathing problems, pain in the forearms and hands
2 Thoracic	heart cardiac valve, coronary vessel	Heart problems
3 Thoracic	Lungs, bronchi, chest	Asthma, bronchitis
4 Thoracic	Gallbladder	Gallbladder problems, shingles
5 Thoracic	Liver, solar plexus, blood	Liver problems, circulatory disturbance, anemia, arthritis
6 Thoracic	Stomach	Stomach problems, heartburn
7 Thoracic	Pancreas, duodenum	Diabetes, heartburn
8 Thoracic	Spleen, diaphragm	Immune deficiency
9 Thoracic	Adrenals	Allergies, eczema
10 Thoracic	Kidneys	Kidney problems, tiredness, calcification of veins
11 Thoracic	Urinary tract	Eczema, acne, urinary problems
12 Thoracic	Small intestine, lymphatic system	Rheumatism, sterility, immune system problems
1 Lumbar	Large intestine, groin	Constipation, colitis
2 Lumbar	Appendix, body, thigh	Appendicitis, varicose veins
3 Lumbar	Ovaries, testicles, bladder, knee	Menstruation problems, impotence
4 Lumbar	Prostate, sciatic nerve	Sciatica, lumbago
5 Lumbar	Lower leg, ankle, toes	Bad circulation in the legs, cramps in the calves
Sacrum	Hip joint, buttocks	Problems in the sacrum and pelvis
Coccyx	Rectum, anus	Pain, hemorrhoids

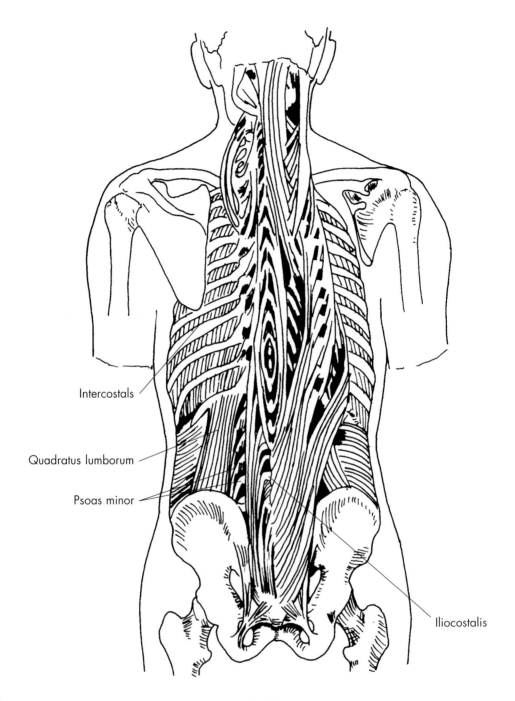

Intercostals

Quadratus lumborum

Psoas minor

Iliocostalis

Fig. 5.18. Back of the tan tien area

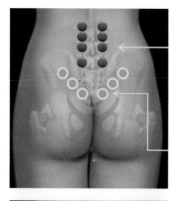

Press the points and grab the shoulder of the other side and loosen points in rotating motion.

Grab points and grab the arm of the other side

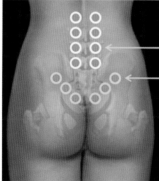

Hold Ming-Men

Joint causes 95% of the Lumbar Spine Pain Syndrom

Fig. 5.19. Ming Men and the Sacrum

The Low Back

From the perspective of the Universal Healing Tao, the lower back is of particular importance because it contains the kidneys, the Ming Men/Door of Life point, and the root of the Microcosmic Orbit (fig. 5.18). It is also the source of pain and discomfort for many thousands of people.

Massage by a trained and knowledgeable Thai massage practitioner can improve the health and functionality of the lower back and the entire spine, rehabilitating the nervous system and therefore aiding the functioning of the body's cells. Thai massage can help deal with vertebra displacement and therefore improve lymph, synovial, and cerebrospinal fluid circulation. This allows the nerves to do their jobs correctly and improves mobility. It also helps deal with pinched nerves in the spine and the pain associated with them.

Evaluating and Treating the Spine

Always use caution when working on the spine; do not treat anyone with severe spinal problems.

1. Palpate down the length of the entire spine, first on one side, then on the other. Try to feel the shape of each vertebra, and also the condition of the tissues between the vertebrae (fig. 5.20).
2. After identifying regions of congestion or inflammation, use one or two fingers to work along the entire spine from top to bottom, massaging away from the bones toward the periphery of the body.

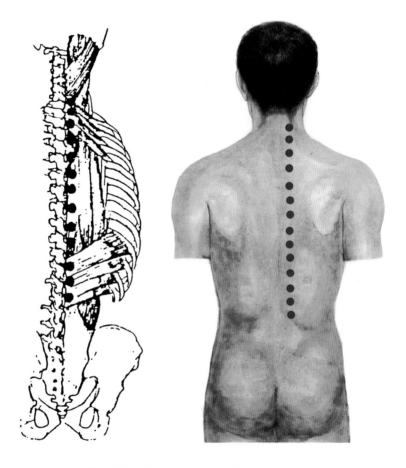

Fig. 5.20. Massage points along the spine

3. Use the heel of your hand to work on the tendinomuscular regions of the Urinary Bladder and Small Intestine channels, then work on any other large areas of tension.
4. Focus on the lower back by holding the Ming Men point with one hand and massaging the sacral points with the other hand (see fig. 5.19 on page 79).
5. Then hold each of the sacral points in turn as you gently pull the opposite arm backward a little bit.

Front of the Torso: The Ribcage

On the front of the body, the internal and external oblique muscles support the rib cage and connect the back to the upper and lower chest (fig. 5.21). The oblique muscles spread out in three different directions, creating a very large and flat muscle region. Because these muscles are generally not visible on the outside, especially with women, palpation is needed to ascertain any tension or problems. The oblique muscles can be felt primarily in the area of the ribs along the side of the torso.

In addition to the obliques, the rectus and transverse abdominis muscles (not shown) also cover and protect the abdominal organs.

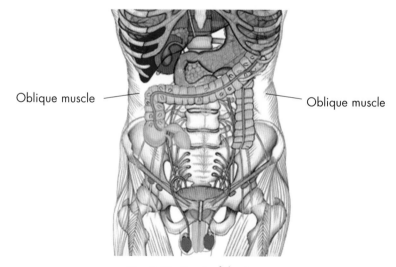

Oblique muscle — Oblique muscle

Fig. 5.21. Front of the torso

Evaluating and Treating the Front of the Torso

1. Have the individual receiving the treatment lie down on his or her back. Place your hands on the person's rib cage and rock the person back and forth slightly. This needs to be done in a relaxed fashion. This gentle but firm movement loosens the muscles in the region. It also helps provide an idea as to where there might be issues with the muscles and tendons.

2. Gently massage the rib cage, working between each rib from the sternum out to the sides. Do not massage directly on the breasts or nipples. Be aware of the many Sen lines and tendinomuscular meridians that run along the chest.

3. Massage along the lower border of the rib cage, feeling the oblique muscles wrapping the torso from back to front.

Front of the Torso: The Navel Region

There are eight distinct regions around the navel (fig. 5.22). These roughly correspond to the eight directions on a compass and reflect

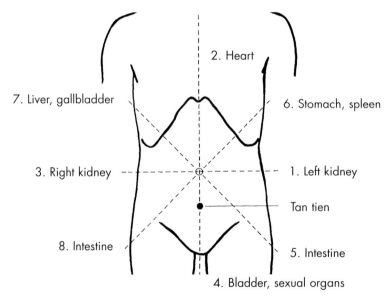

Fig. 5.22. Eight points around the navel correspond to the internal organs.

the health of the major organs. While the careful evaluation and massage of the organs is discussed in detail in our books *Chi Nei Tsang* and *Advanced Chi Nei Tsang,** this volume will primarily address the prominent muscles and tendons of this region.

Massaging the Navel Region

You can perform this massage on yourself as well as others.

1. Using one or two fingers, create tight spirals as you work around the navel in a clockwise direction (fig. 5.23).

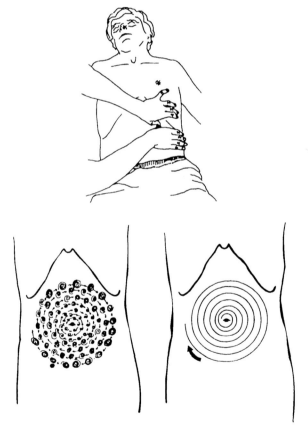

Fig. 5.23. Create tight spirals. Move in clockwise circles beginning at the navel; gradually spiral out toward the perimeter of the abdomen.

---

*Mantak Chia, *Chi Nei Tsang* (Rochester, Vt.: Destiny Books, 2007) and Mantak Chia, *Advanced Chi Nei Tsang* (Rochester, Vt.: Destiny Books, 2009).

2. Continue to spiral outward toward the perimeter of the abdomen.
3. Next, place one hand on top of the other and use the heel of your bottom hand to massage the abdomen around the navel. This area is a tender portion of the body and caution should be used. Apply downward pressure as your student pushes his abdomen upward using the abdominal muscles.

This massage activates the tendons in the abdominal region, and especially the organ tendons. In addition, it activates the veins and arteries.

A breathing technique can be used to help expand the energy and power of the tendons. Concentrating on the abdominal area, a person inhales and expands the tendons and then exhales and allows the tendons to return. This should be done with a relaxed approach that brings about a feeling of well-being. Breathe in and then out in an almost meditative fashion. Strengthening the tendons helps one feel and actually be younger relative to one's overall health.

The Abdominal Organs

When massaging the front of the trunk, it is helpful to know something about the internal organs that may be affected by the massage (fig. 5.24). According to the principles of Chinese medicine, these organs govern many internal body functions; improving stagnation and releasing blockages that affect these organs can thus affect the health profoundly.

The liver is located on the righthand side of the abdomen over the gallbladder. This organ is associated with the gallbladder, the wood element, spring, the color green, the sour flavor, the eyes, and vision, as well as with emotional well-being, anger, aggression, kindness, and forgiveness.

Imbalances in the liver can lead to muscle and tendon tightness, emotional outbursts, menstrual irregularities, and headaches, among other issues.

The spleen is located in the upper left part of the abdomen, beneath the rib cage. The spleen is associated with the earth element, the stomach, the sweet flavor, digestion, the mouth, Indian summer, and the color yellow, as well as with worry, compassion, balance, and openness.

Imbalances in the spleen can lead to digestive problems, bleeding disorders, fatigue, and weakness, among other issues.

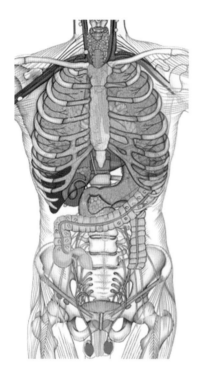

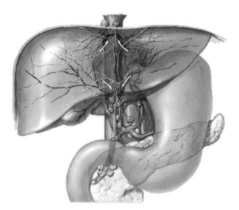

Fig. 5.24. Be aware of the abdominal organs as you massage the front of the torso.

The kidneys and the tan tien. While the kidneys are closer to the back of the body than the front, abdominal massage will affect both the kidneys and the tan tien. The kidneys are associated with the water element, the urinary bladder, winter, the color blue, and the salty flavor, as well as with sexual energy, the ears, hearing, the bones, fear, and courage.

Imbalances in the kidneys can lead to a host of problems including fatigue, lack of sexual energy, and lack of will power. An imbalanced tan tien can lead to breathing problems, posture issues, and difficulties with balance and movement.

The Psoas Muscles

The psoas muscles, long muscles on each side of the lumbar region, are like a bridge from the upper portion of the body to the lower part (fig. 5.25). The psoas is involved in flexing the leg up toward the body and helps maintain the structure of the hips, pelvis, and lower back. The psoas can also influence standing or walking.

A good way to discover these muscle is to sit for a long period, which allows the psoas muscles to shorten. When you stand up again, you will feel contracted and tight in the pelvis and hips.

When one of the psoas muscles is too tight or short on one side, a tilting in the vertebrae results, which can cause back pain in some individuals. Other postural problems that can be caused by tight psoas muscles are compressed vertebrae, bad posture, hip or leg pain, and a protruding abdomen. Figure 5.26 shows some of the important relationships of the psoas to other parts of the body.

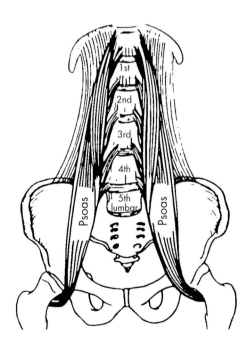

Fig. 5.25. Psoas muscles

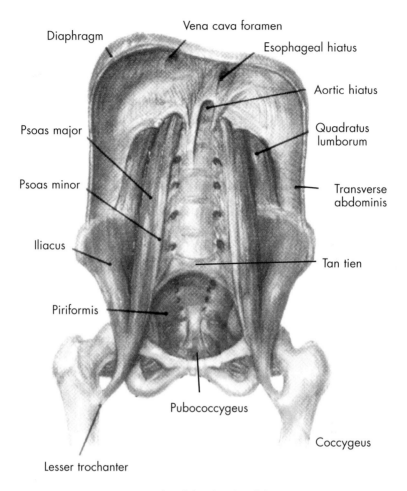

Diaphragm

Vena cava foramen

Esophageal hiatus

Aortic hiatus

Psoas major

Quadratus lumborum

Psoas minor

Transverse abdominis

Iliacus

Tan tien

Piriformis

Pubococcygeus

Coccygeus

Lesser trochanter

Fig. 5.26. Front side of the "back" of the tan tien

In addition to their influence on posture, the psoas muscles also affect the tan tien, the kidneys, the sexual organs, and the intestines. In fact, the psoas muscle system (see fig. 5.27 on page 88) can be understood as a supporting shelf below the kidneys in the back of the tan tien; this support helps to keep the kidneys happy and secure (see fig. 5.28 on page 88).

The psoas also responds to emotions in the kidneys, however. Fear, for example, which can create cold in the kidneys, also precipitates a tightening and shortening of the psoas.

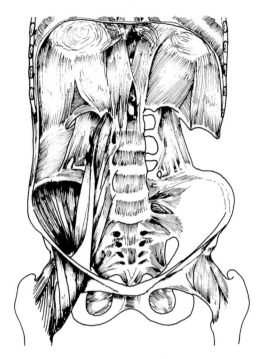

Fig. 5.27. Psoas muscle system

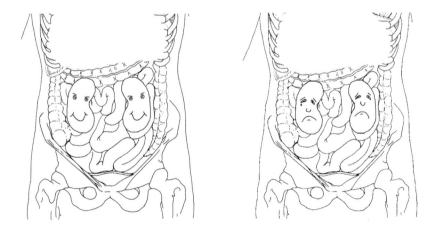

Fig. 5.28. Kidney emotions affect the psoas muscle

Releasing the Psoas Muscles

It is important to work on the psoas because of its close relationship to the kidneys, sexual energy, solar plexus, nerves, and many blood vessels in this area. When the psoas is held in contraction, the free flow of sexual energy is disrupted. Maintaining the psoas releases energy into the organs and legs, and balances the tan tien, which helps to activate the chi.

1. Locate the psoas muscles on each side by asking your student to raise one knee up to the chest. Ask the student to rotate the knee back and forth; this movement will engage the psoas muscle on this side and help you to find it.
2. When you feel the psoas contract, press your finger pads deeply into the body until you reach it (fig. 5.29). While your finger pads

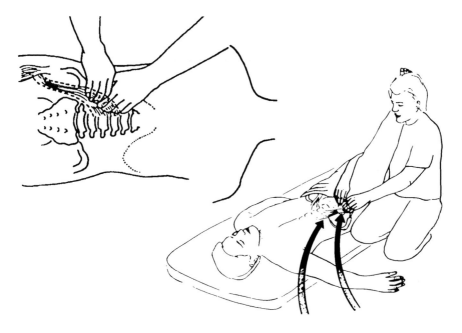

Fig. 5.29. Releasing the psoas muscles

press down to the depth of the psoas, you can line your individual fingers up along its length.

3. Continue pressing down and feel for any excessive contractions. You may also feel a spiraling contraction. When there has been excessive fear, the psoas often responds by contracting with a spiraling force. Maintain your deep pressure and slowly move the pads of your fingers in a lateral direction, unwinding the spiraling force and tension of the psoas.

4. Continue with this pressure and lateral movement, slowly working the full length of the psoas.

5. Repeat on the other side.

You—and your students—can maintain your psoas muscles in good condition by practicing the Universal Healing Tao's Tao Yin exercises.* These practices focus on growing the tendons, relaxing the psoas muscle and the diaphragm, and developing strength and flexibility in the body.

The Genital Area

This sensitive area has many links to a person's body, mind, spirit, and emotions (fig. 5.30). Take special care and communicate clearly with your student when working on this part of the body.

The circulation system of the genitals is greatly affected when the inguinal ligaments are overly contracted. When the inguinal ligaments are shortened from poor alignment or other causes, the fascial tissue will also tighten and shorten. This will then affect the blood flow and lymphatic flow into and out of the genitals.

---

*See Mantak Chia, *Energy Balance through the Tao* (Rochester, Vt.: Destiny Books, 2005), 59–82.

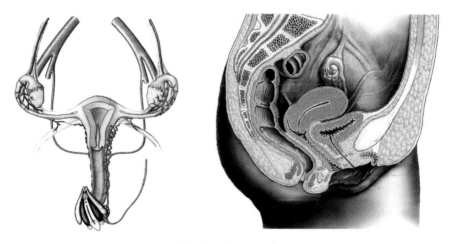

Fig. 5.30. Female genital areas

 Releasing the Inguinal Ligament

Because the energy channels flow through the tendons, ligaments, and meridians, it is possible to treat issues pertaining to the genitals of both males and females.

1. Using the pads of your fingers or the outside of your thumb, press into the base of the inguinal ligament where it attaches at the pubic bone (fig. 5.31). Slowly move your hand up along the

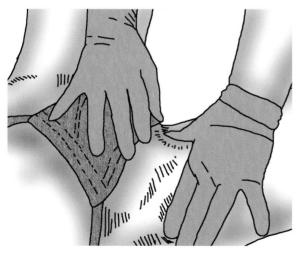

Fig. 5.31. Releasing the inguinal ligament

ligament, feeling it lengthen under your touch until you reach its attachment at the crest of the pelvis. Repeat this movement a few times until you feel the ligament soften and relax.

2. Repeat on the other side.

 ## Releasing the Inner Thigh

1. Move a little away from your student and rotate the left leg exteriorly so that the inside of the leg is exposed. In this position the gracilis and adductor muscles will contract and bulge out a bit.
2. Place your left hand over the genitals and stabilize them to the left.
3. Press into the left leg with your right thumb (fig. 5.32); begin underneath the bulging muscles and to the outside of the genitals, and massage with a long stroke down the inside of the leg. Repeat these movements until you feel a softening in the muscles and the leg release.
4. Repeat on the inside of the right leg.

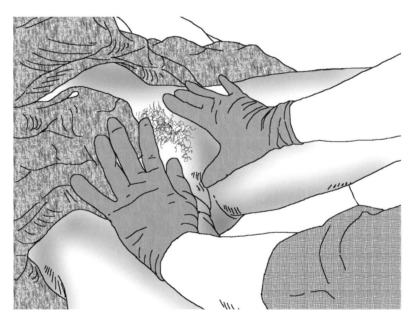

Fig. 5.32. Releasing the inner thigh

Hips

The hips act as a bridge between the spine and the legs. Essentially, they connect the upper body with the lower extremities (fig. 5.33). The hips support the weight of the body and they are indispensable for maintaining balance while standing upright.

The bony hips have many ligaments that facilitate stability and smooth movement (see fig. 5.34 on page 94). Massaging the hip area helps to keep these ligaments healthy and elastic.

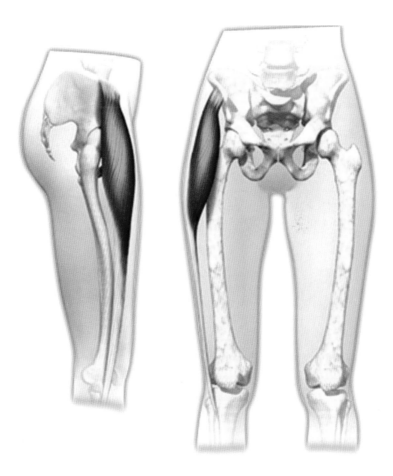

Fig. 5.33. The hips

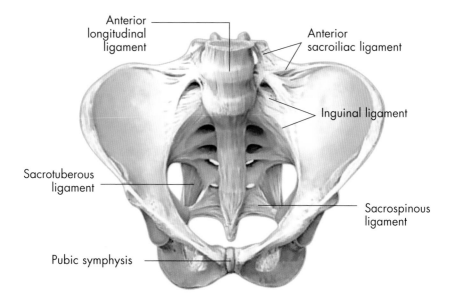

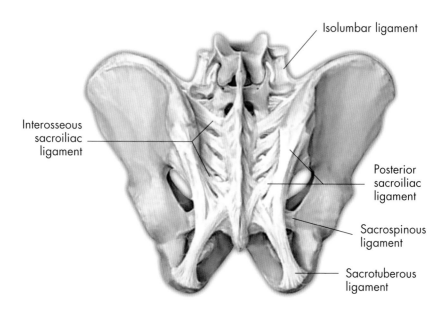

Fig. 5.34. Ligaments of the hip (anterior and posterior views)

Muscles Involved in Hip Movement

Hip movement requires coordinated activity from the muscles of the trunk, buttocks, and thighs—primarily the iliopsoas, rectus femoris, and tensor fasciae latae in the front, and the gluteus medius and maximus in the back (fig. 5.35).

One of the most important hip muscles is the piriformis, which lies deep under the gluteus muscles and connects the sacrum to the greater trochanter of the hip (fig. 5.36).

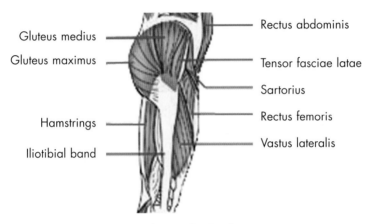

Fig. 5.35. Muscles involved in hip movement

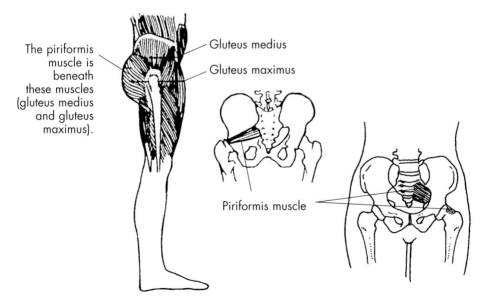

Fig. 5.36. The piriformis muscle connects the hip to the sacrum.

Because many hip problems originate with tightness or spasm in the piriformis and iliopsoas muscles, massage of these two muscles is the primary focus of work in the hip region.

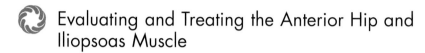 Evaluating and Treating the Anterior Hip and Iliopsoas Muscle

1. Have your student lie on the treatment table with his buttocks on the table and legs hanging down toward the floor.
2. Have the student raise his right leg up and down as you palpate the front of the hip, feeling the main muscles and tendons for tension and armoring.
3. Press into any tense areas as the student continues slowly raising and lowering the leg you are working on.

Massaging the Iliopsoas Muscle

The iliacus muscle joins the psoas muscle in the lateral wall of the pelvis to become the iliopsoas muscle. The iliopsoas is the most powerful flexor of the leg at the hip joint, and when this muscle is held in flexion it disrupts the circulation and flow of energy in the genital area.

1. On the right hip, press with your right thumb into the inside curve of your student's right pelvic crest (the anterior, superior iliac spine) (fig. 5.37). Place the rest of your right hand around the

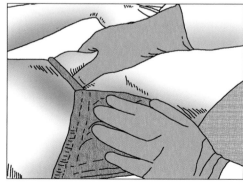

Fig. 5.37. Massaging the iliacus muscle and iliac crest

back side of the pelvis for stabilization. When you work on your student's right hip, use your left hand to stabilize and massage.

2. Move your right thumb into the inside curve and follow the edge of the ileum, massaging the ligaments attached to the iliac crest and the iliacus muscle. Feel for a softening and an increase of space in this area.

Evaluating and Treating the Posterior Hip and Piriformis Muscle

Evaluate the posterior hip the same way you did the front, by having your student raise and lower her legs as you palpate the muscles and tendons around the hip joint.

1. Have your student lie face down on the treatment table, with her legs dangling toward the floor.
2. Palpate the muscles and tendons as the student slowly raises and lowers her leg; press and hold tight or tense areas while the movement continues.

Massaging the Piriformis Muscle

1. Place the student on his or her left side. Feel for an indentation or "hole" between the gluteus medius and gluteus maximus to find the piriformis muscle (see fig. 5.36 on page 95).
2. Press straight down with your thumb or elbow to massage and release the contracted piriformis muscle (see fig. 5.38 on page 98). Often this area is very painful, especially if there is a sciatic problem.

While the massage can be painful, it has a "sweet ache" to it; it hurts, but the student starts to feel that he or she is going to get better. Do not forget to use your concentration to send healing energy into this area.

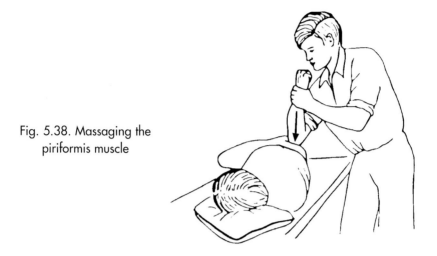

Fig. 5.38. Massaging the
piriformis muscle

Legs

All of the tendons and ligaments in the leg support the weight of the
body and are critical for movement. The leg muscles are the strongest
muscles in the body, while the Achilles tendon is the strongest tendon
in the body (fig. 5.39).

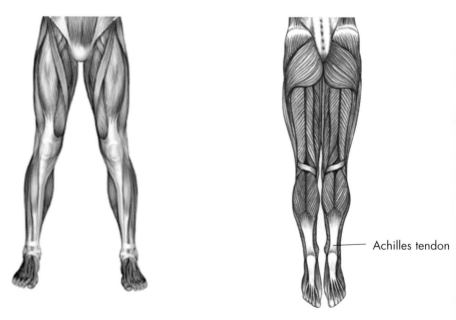

Achilles tendon

Fig. 5.39. Muscles and tendons in the legs, front and rear view

Many issues with the legs, arms, or other parts of the body are the result of tendons being too tight; when they wrap around the bones they direct energy flow upward. Muscles and tendons that are too tight pull everything and have a negative impact on our health and mobility. If this happens in one leg, it can make that leg "shorter" than the other leg and tilt the entire body.

Evaluating and Treating the Upper Leg

1. Have your student lie on her back on the treatment table, with one leg extended and one knee up.
2. Hold the ankle and calf of the bent leg with one hand and place your other hand on the thigh muscles.
3. Slowly slide the foot forward, palpating the thigh as the leg extends. The thigh muscles may be rigid or tight, and the client may find this stretch painful.
4. Press and hold any areas of tension, then massage with appropriate Chi Nei Tsang strokes.

Releasing Tendons in the Upper Leg

The purpose of this treatment is to release tendons that are "stuck" to the bone, so that the information that is held in them can be released. If the tendons are tight, the blood flow is obstructed. The tendons of the upper leg need to be loosened so that everything functions properly.

1. Begin with the person receiving the massage lying on his or her back with one knee bent up to a 45-degree angle. The sole of the foot of the bent leg should be flat against the table.
2. Hold the inside of the leg and ask the person to push inward, then release, then push again. This should be repeated several times while you press around the hip and groin area to feel the tendons.
3. Press and hold any areas of tension, then massage with appropriate Chi Nei Tsang strokes.

4. Repeat steps 2 and 3 while holding the outside of the knee and having the person push against the resistance.

Knee

The tendons and ligaments of the knee joint are vulnerable to strains and tears—especially among athletes (fig. 5.40). Because such injuries are more likely when the tendons are tight, regular stretching and massage treatment of legs can help to prevent them.

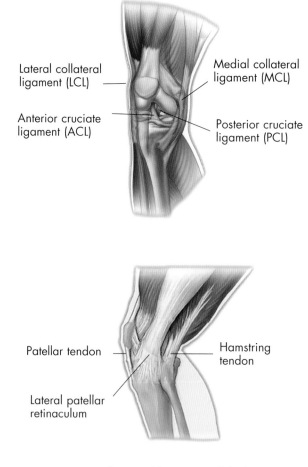

Lateral collateral ligament (LCL)

Medial collateral ligament (MCL)

Anterior cruciate ligament (ACL)

Posterior cruciate ligament (PCL)

Patellar tendon

Hamstring tendon

Lateral patellar retinaculum

Fig. 5.40. Tendons and ligaments of the knee

Figure 5.41 below shows how the tendons can wrap around the bone as the result of the knee being twisted outward.

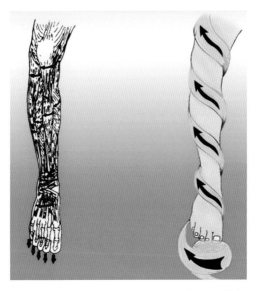

Fig. 5.41. Tendon wrap: when the knee is twisted out, all the tendons wrap around the bone, directing the energy flow upward.

 Releasing Tendons in the Knee Joint

The object of this technique is to release tendons that are stuck on the bone. If done properly, the practitioner will be able to feel the tendons. As is the case with all bones, palpation and treatment never consists of applying pressure or tapping directly on the knee. Rather, it is done around the knee cap moving in an outward motion. Treatment releases the flow of energy that has been blocked by stress/injury.

1. Begin with the person receiving the massage lying on his or her back with one knee bent up to a 45-degree angle. The sole of the foot on the bent leg should be flat against the table.
2. Place your hand behind the middle of the person's bent knee and have the person slowly slide the leg down to a flat position, then back up to bent. Take care this is not done too quickly.

3. While the person moves his or her leg downward and upward, wrap your hand around the knee and use your fingers to palpate the area. Repeat the downward and upward motion three times.

4. Then slide your hand to a lower position behind the knee and repeat the procedure.

5. Use Chi Nei Tsang strokes to massage all around the knee. Focus on any areas of tightness, and pay special attention to the points as illustrated below (fig. 5.42).

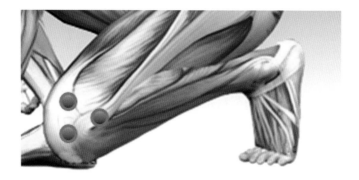

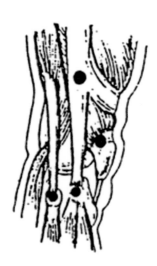

Fig. 5.42. Points on the knee

Releasing the Back of the Knee

1. Massage down the back of the thigh to loosen the muscles there.
2. Next, massage the points on the back of the knee as shown in figure 5.43 below.

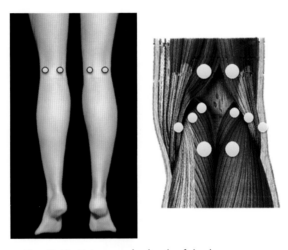

Fig. 5.43. Points on the back of the knee

3. Next, hold the knee as shown in figure 5.44 below, grasping the popliteal tendons behind the leg.
4. Massage with your thumbs on the left and right sides of the tendons, using your fingers to pull them apart.

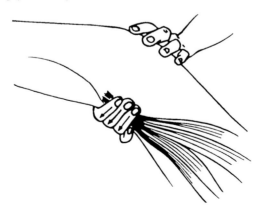

Fig. 5.44. Grasp the popliteal tendons and muscles.

The Lower Leg and Ankle

The muscles and tendons of the lower leg are activated as the foot is placed on the ground, and as it pushes off (fig. 5.45). When the legs are in good condition, these tendons and muscles feel springy and alive. When they become stiff, our balance and movement become more difficult.

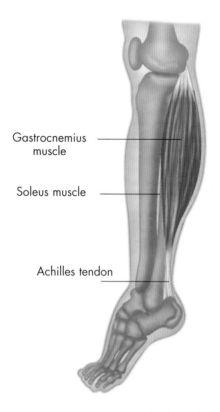

Gastrocnemius muscle

Soleus muscle

Achilles tendon

Fig. 5.45. The lower leg

The tendons and ligaments of the ankle are quite vulnerable to strains and injuries; the impacts of jumps, falls, and missteps are most likely to reveal themselves in this region (fig. 5.46). Women who wear high heels place added strain on their feet, ankles, legs, and low backs.

The ankle can be a problem for anyone, depending on how they walk. However, it can particularly be a problem for women who

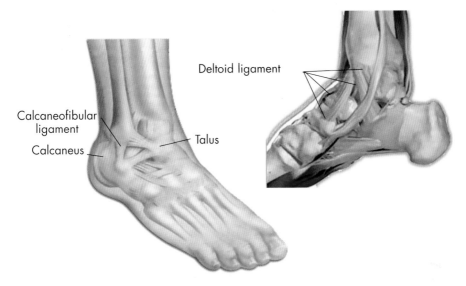

Deltoid ligament

Calcaneofibular
ligament

Talus

Calcaneus

Fig. 5.46. Ligaments and tendons of the ankle

wear high heels. Ankle problems can be very painful. The first thing to look for is where the individual's gait twists. An examination of the ankle is necessary. If the twisting is to the inside, the outside of the ankle suffers. If the twisting is to the outside, the inside of the ankle suffers. The keys to problems are the tendons that attach to the anklebone.

Evaluating and Treating the Ankle

1. Rotate the ankle in a turning type motion as you palpate the major tendons. Feel for any areas of stiffness, and ask your student to point out any areas of pain.
2. Next, continue palpating around the ankle as you push the foot downward from the toe and then release it.
3. Massage all around the tendons and ligaments of the ankle, using your fingertips or knuckles.
4. Continue palpating and massaging until the tension and pain have released.

Feet

The human foot contains numerous joints, bones, tendons, ligaments, and muscles (fig. 5.47). These assist with motion as well as balance. As they work, the tendons of the feet release stored up energy, which is essential for walking and running. For example, when a person walks, energy flows outward as he steps and presses the toe slightly downward. Foot tendons are very complicated and, in the event that they break, it takes a long period of time for them to heal.

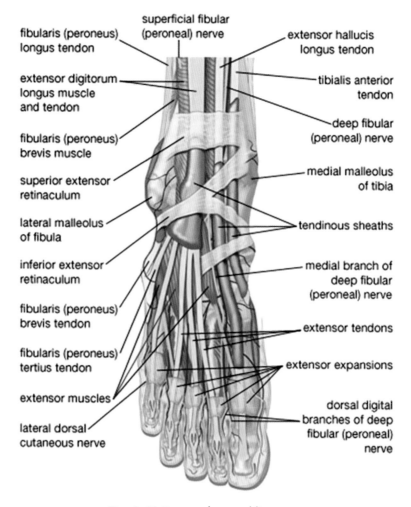

Fig. 5.47. Foot tendons and ligaments

In human beings, part of the function of the feet is to allow an upright posture. While this is very useful much of the time, it also happens to result in a great deal of stress and strain on the feet and ankles. Anyone who has had a problem in this region of the body, or even followed sports, is aware of the difficulties that can come about in the event of injury to the feet or ankles. Some of the painful issues that can develop in the feet are arthritis, plantar fasciitis, bunions, Achilles tendon injury, and gout.

The sole of the foot is the part of the body that directly touches the earth. Issues of balance and grounding can often affect the health and function of the sole, which contains the important acupuncture point known as Bubbling Spring.

Traditional Thai massage of the feet, like that of other areas of the body, increases flexibility by releasing blockages that can cause stiffness and other issues. It also helps facilitate the removal of toxins in the circulatory system and energy channels, rejuvenating the body as well as the mind and spirit. There are many benefits to such treatment, including increased energy, reduced pain, better relaxation, stress relief, and improved sleep, as well as increased performance and endurance in athletes.

Stretching and Activating the Feet

The therapist can activate the tendons throughout the leg and, indeed, the entire body, using the foot.

1. Have your student lie face up on a mat or massage table. Push against the bottom of his feet near the toes, as he pushes back against your hand.

2. Next, have your student stand on a mat and stretch one foot at a time by pressing the pads of the toes into the mat while lifting the heel up to a vertical angle (roughly 90 degrees). This results in a downward push in the toes that is felt as a backward push in the heels.

These exercises give a good stretch to the ligaments, tendons, and muscles in the toes and bottoms of the feet, and they stimulate the Bubbling Springs point. Further, they engage the Achilles tendon and the backs of the legs.

 ## Massaging the Feet

Before massaging the feet, it is a good idea to perform the tendon stretches from the exercise above.

1. Massage the tendons and ligaments of the feet with your finger-tips, working along the tops of the feet from the ankle toward the toes (see fig. 5.47 on page 106).
2. Next, work the tendons of the toes (fig. 5.48) by slowly twisting each toe and then releasing it. Twist, then release, twist and release, repeating until the tendons are looser.
3. Massage the Bubbling Spring point with your thumb or, as shown in figure 5.49, with your elbow. Apply pressure to the point for about 30 seconds and then release.
4. Massage the other acupressure points as shown in figure 5.50.

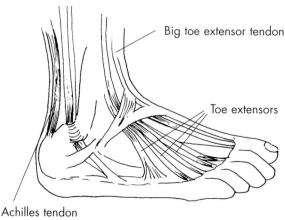

Fig. 5.48. Foot tendons

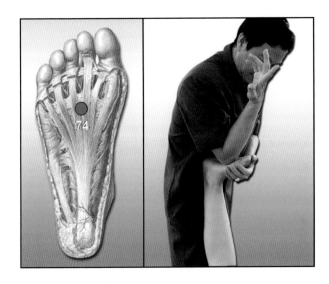

Fig. 5.49. Bubbling Spring point

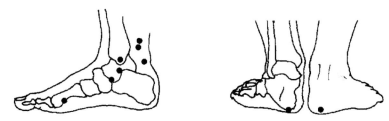

Fig. 5.50. Chi Nei Tsang massage points on the feet

Foot massage therapy is an excellent practice for relief of stressed and sore feet, and it is also deeply healing because the regions of the feet correspond to other areas of the body. With this in mind, the therapist utilizes various acupressure points in the foot to treat assorted maladies in conjunction with their corresponding organs. Among the health issues that are related to the foot are insomnia, headache, and high blood pressure.

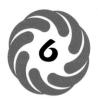

Traditional Tok Sen

Tok Sen is a unique healing modality found only in the Lanna region of Thailand—the area around Chiang Mai in the north. The practice sends mechanical and sound vibrations deep into the fascia, tendons, and muscles to clear blocked energy from the channels in the body. "Tok" means to "clear" or "take off," while "Sen" denotes the Sen lines. Tok Sen is thought to date back over five thousand years, developing in Thailand while acupuncture developed in China. Having been handed down orally from generation to generation, this energy healing method is still practiced in rural areas. Tok Sen helps to improve energy flow, relieve aching muscles, and maintain healthy tendons.

As mentioned elsewhere, traditional Thai medicine views the body as a whole and emphasizes the connection between things. Another way of thinking of this is that one part of the body communicates with other parts of the body. In addition, the body communicates with its surroundings. Blockages and stagnation can impair these modes of communication, thereby causing imbalances and illness. Tok Sen deals with these imbalances by treating the avenues of communication—the energy lines. Once the energy blockage or imbalance is dealt with, healing can take place. It should be noted that a knowledgeable practitioner has a special wisdom relative to the human body and maintains a connection that is both physical and spiritual to the person being treated.

By tapping the body using traditional Tok Sen tools—a wooden hammer and variety of pestles—vibrations are sent through the nerves, muscles, and fascia to treat muscle and tendon pain (fig. 6.1). A light "hammering" with varying degrees of contact is applied to the different regions of the body. Of course, the tools are never applied in a violent or rough manner. The vibrations created by the gentle hammering work deeply into the fascia and muscles, repairing and rejuvenating them, and making them feel more alive. Among the many advantages of Tok Sen treatment is the fact that some muscles are too big or too deep for the fingers to reach. Tok Sen, on the other hand, can penetrate to those regions. Furthermore, the smaller and thinner pestles can get into small areas that the fingers cannot effectively reach.

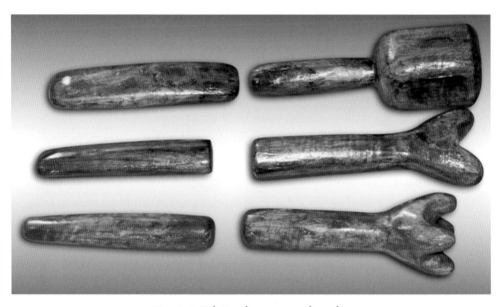

Fig. 6.1. Tok Sen hammer and pestles

Knowledgeable practitioners will use their fingers and hands as supplements to the treatment—as a means of checking the areas that have been treated in order to measure how successful the work has been and whether additional treatment is needed.

TOK SEN BENEFITS

Just a few of the advantages of this ancient Thai treatment are increased circulation, relief from stiff and tight muscles, and improvement of nerve functions. In addition, many maladies that decrease the quality of life can be improved with Tok Sen.

The main function of this treatment relates to the tendons and specifically to the tendinomuscular meridians. The vibration of the tendons, when done correctly, loosens both the tendons and the muscles. It also improves the blood circulation. In traditional Thai medicine, many problems are caused by blood vessels that "cling" too rigidly to the bones, becoming inflexible. Tok Sen is excellent for treating this problem and the issues accompanying it.

Because it treats the body in a holistic manner, Tok Sen therapy can have a wide range of benefits, as shown in the list below.

1. Increases blood circulation. Better circulation nourishes tendons and releases blocked energy more quickly.
2. Relaxes muscles. Tight muscles will squeeze capillaries, which decreases blood circulation to muscles and causes muscle soreness. Hammering on the meridians assists in relieving pain and discomfort. This is especially true if a person has stored a lot of stress and created a hard or armored shell on the tendons and muscles.
3. Stimulates peripheral nerves. These nerves run parallel with capillaries. Every time we hammer, the vibration will nourish capillaries and peripheral nerves, which can stimulate muscles as well.
4. Releases pain from many causes:
   • Headaches from nerve problems, migraines, brain degeneration, blurred vision, or hearing loss
   • Shoulder pain, neck sprain, shoulder tendon tightness, immobile arm
   • Tendon compression, back muscle tightness, scapular problems, and back pain

- Lower back pain, spinal cord inflammation, difficulty bending the trunk
- Lumbar pain and nerve compression
- Thigh pain, hamstring muscle tightness, and patella dislocation
- Calf pain, sole pain, and numbness
- Arm pain, elbow pain, arm numbness, and hand numbness.

TOK SEN TOOLS

The healing vibrations are created by the tapping of the Tok Sen tools. The treatment does not involve hard striking but more of a tapping, directed to specific areas depending on the condition being treated. The tapping of a pestle is usually done in a repeated tempo of three strokes.

The quality and integrity of the tools is important for the practitioner. These tools are traditionally made from wood of the tamarind tree, although other materials can be used and these also result in highly effective treatment. Wood is especially good at transmitting vibrations into the nerves and muscles.

The Tok Sen Hammer

The Tok Sen wooden hammer has a rectangular head of about 4 inches in length, with a perimeter of about 2.5 inches. It has a rounded handle about 6 inches long. The use of the hammer is obvious. It is

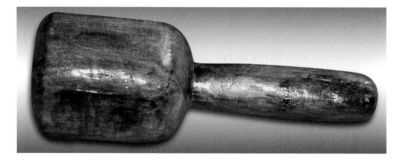

Fig. 6.2. Tok Sen hammer

used to tap the pestle, which sends healing vibrations into the tendons and muscles. These vibrations help to release the tendons, blood vessels, and energy channels that are "stuck" to the bones. They also help to loosen and release information from significant meridians in the body.

The Tok Sen Pestles

The five common pestles—also called "wedges"—are applied to distinct parts of the body. The smaller wedges are for areas that are tighter, while the bigger pestles are used in the case of large muscles, for example. The wedges must be placed at the correct angle and tapped three or four times. The practitioner then moves the pestle slightly while continuing to tap.

> **The circle wedge** is used for tapping on large tendons in the neck and body.
>
> **The smaller flat wedge** is usually the most frequently employed by the practitioner because it can be used almost anywhere on the body. It particularly assists in releasing tendons caught between bones in the shoulders, arms, and legs. It can penetrate deeply into the tendinomuscular meridians to relieve pains in the large joints.
>
> **The larger flat wedge** is useful on the bottoms of the feet and palms of the hands.
>
> **The two-legged knocker** is used for tapping in two areas simultaneously, such as between two bones or on two muscles. It is most commonly used along the spinal cord and around small bones.
>
> **The four-legged knocker** is used for the sacrum and other areas that are appropriate.

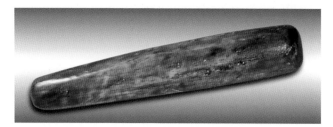

Fig. 6.3.
Circle wedge

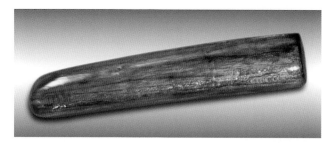

Fig. 6.4. Small
flat wedge

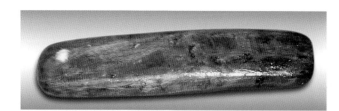

Fig. 6.5. Large
flat wedge

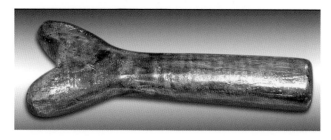

Fig. 6.6. Two-
legged knocker

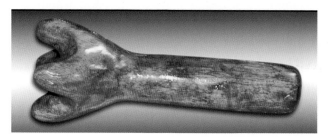

Fig. 6.7. Four-
legged knocker

As the tools are used on many people, they need to be cleaned after each therapy session. Generally this can be done with soap and water, a rinsing, and a thorough drying. An additional method is to wipe the tools with alcohol, which sterilizes the instruments and dries quickly so that the wood is not adversely affected. As with all things, care and attention to even these details will have an influence on the practitioner as well as the treatment.

GENERAL GUIDELINES FOR TOK SEN TREATMENT

When practicing Tok Sen, it is important to keep the following general principles in mind.

Positioning

Tok Sen can be performed with the client assuming any of the following positions, depending on the condition and the area being worked:

1. Supine
2. Prone
3. Side-lying
4. Sitting

Working with the Pestles

A few general rules apply to working with the pestles, which are unique to Tok Sen practice.

1. A small amount of mild herbal oil can be used to help the pestle slide easily along the skin.
2. Always remember that the tapping of the pestles with the hammer is never applied directly to any bone.

3. Different pestles might be needed for different people. For example, the four-legged knocker might be better on the spinal cord of smaller individuals.

4. The pestle is generally used at a slight angle to the side of the bone, relative to the position of the person receiving the treatment.

The Importance of Palpation

Touching an area and a bit of common sense allows you to know which pestle to use. Of course this is also true of knowing exactly where to apply the treatment. The more experience you have, the more your fingers have developed the ability to "know" what they are touching.

Patience

Patience and attention to detail is required on the part of the practitioner. In addition, however, the individual being treated must exercise patience: each treatment requires at least one hour, and often two. Treating the legs alone can sometimes take one hour. Additional patience is required because the benefits of Tok Sen therapy are generally not instantaneous and often require more than one treatment. Furthermore, maintenance treatments are usually required.

PROTOCOLS FOR TREATING SPECIFIC AILMENTS WITH TOK SEN

Many conditions can be helped using this ancient Thai therapy. These include everything from muscular and tendon problems all the way to troubles pertaining to the organs of the body. The Tok Sen practitioner uses knowledge of the energy lines in the body to release the energy that is blocked. Depending on what indications and issues are involved, treatment using traditional massage might be incorporated into the overall plan as well.

Here is a list of some treatment protocols for Tok Sen, for issues ranging over a number of aspects and functions of the body from head to toe.

TOK SEN TREATMENT PROTOCOLS

INDICATION	TREATMENT METHOD
Dizziness and headache	Hammer at occipital area.
Headache	Hammer in front of knees.
Dry mouth	Hammer at malleolus up through knee, thigh, and breast.
Stiff neck	Hammer at paravertebral muscles (neck to lumbar).
Chest pain	Hammer at chest.
Chest swelling	Hammer at breast.
Scapular pain	Hammer at chest below clavicle.
Shoulder pain	Hammer neck, arms, and shoulders.
Elbow syndrome	Hammer at elbow.
Hand syndrome	Hammer at arms and shoulders.
Hand numbness	Hammer at arms and shoulders.
Fingertip numbness or pain	Hammer at right and left breast.
Muscle tightness	Hammer at side of foot.
Trunk tightness	Hammer from shoulder to hand and abdomen.
Trunk muscles stiff	Hammer at sacrum.
Back pain down through both legs and numbness to tip of toes	Check nerve compression, hammer lumbar area and hips.
Back and leg muscles tight	Treat in prone position.
Lower back pain from kidney problem	Do not hammer; if problem is *not* caused by kidney problem, hammering is allowed.
Lumbar problems	Hammer at lumbar spine.
Knee pain from bone spur or swelling	Don't hammer.
Stiff knees and legs	Hammer at malleolus up through sides of knees.
Shin problems	Hammer from knees to thighs.
Foot swelling	Hammer at thigh close to sexual organs.

INDICATION	TREATMENT METHOD
Foot tightness and stiffness	Hammer at lumbar spine down through thighs, knees, and shins.
Feeling hot at the soles of the feet	Hammer at middle of calf on lateral side.
Frequent urination	Hammer at top of thigh to middle of thigh.
Urinary incontinence	Hammer at tendons close to sacrum.
Hemiplegia and paraplegia	Hammer below malleolus.
Blood detoxification	Hammer at calf.
Pain from muscle knots, numbness, trigger fingers, inability to grasp	Use large flat wedge; hammer until pain decreases.

TOK SEN TREATMENT, SUPINE POSITION

A general Tok Sen treatment often begins with the patient in a supine position, with treatment of the navel region, abdomen, and chest.

Treating the Front of the Torso: The Navel Area, Upper Abdomen, and Chest

Hammering around the Navel

One of the primary focal points in Tok Sen—as in many Eastern medical practices—is the area around the navel. This area is crucial because of its relationship with the internal organs and energy channels throughout the body. Proper treatment of the region surrounding the navel releases stress and tension from the organs and helps the channels let go of negative emotions that have collected there, allowing excessive accumulation of blood and other life forces to be released.

1. Beginning with the small flat wedge, hammer the tendons directly around the navel (see fig. 6.8 on page 120). Tap in a rhythm of three strokes, then slide the pestle a little bit and tap rhythmically again. Continue working around the navel in widening spirals, feeling the vibrations going into the tendons. Where tension is felt, harder tapping can be done. Be aware of the starting points of the Sen Sib (see fig. 6.9 on page 120) as you work in this area.

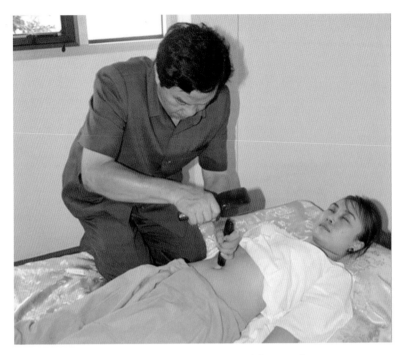

Fig. 6.8. Hammering around the navel

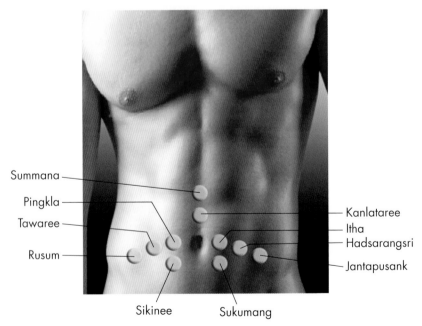

Fig. 6.9. Sen Sib starting points

2. Next, tap the area under the navel, angling and sliding the small pestle downward as shown in figure 6.10.

3. Next, tap the lines at the bottom of the rib cage, beginning at the center and working outward. For reference, it is helpful to understand how this area reflects and releases the winds from the individual organs (fig. 6.11).

4. Palpate the abdomen to check for any remaining tension. Repeat any areas if necessary.

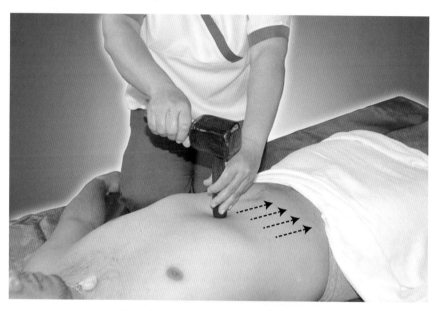

Fig. 6.10. Hammering the abdomen

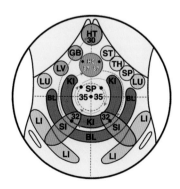

Fig. 6.11. Be aware of the organs associated with each area of the abdomen.

◉ Hammering the Chest

The area of the chest includes the rib cage and extends up to the shoulders. Among the benefits from treatment to this area is the opening of the lungs. Some patients will quickly notice an improvement in their breathing, and it is of particular help to those who suffer from asthma. It is also good for the heart, loosening the tendons beneath it, which can help prevent heart attacks.

Of course, treatment of the chest also benefits the circulatory system. Negative particles, including heavy metals, can cause obstructions in the circulatory system and accumulate in the organs. Tok Sen can assist in removing such obstructions.

1. Palpate the rib cage area and rock it back and forth a bit to discern where the areas of tightness are. Plan to work a little more intensively in the tighter areas.
2. Beginning beneath the clavicle on either side, tap the small pestle in a slow, rhythmic motion. Angle the pestle directly downward, then outward toward the arm. You are simultaneously tapping and slowly sliding the pestle outward. The tapping is done lightly and carefully, treating the tendons, muscles, and nerves (fig. 6.12).

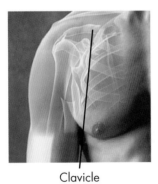

Clavicle

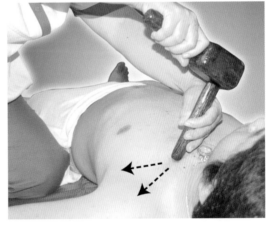

Fig. 6.12. Hammering the chest

3. Work your way down the ribcage, placing the pestle between each pair of ribs, then tapping lightly and sliding outward (fig. 6.13).
4. Repeat steps 2 and 3 on the other side of the chest.
5. Palpate the chest region again, to see if any area needs further treatment, and repeat the steps as necessary.

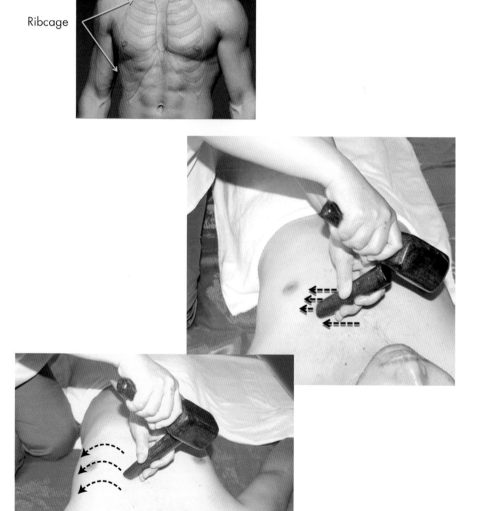

Ribcage

Fig. 6.13. Hammering between the ribs

Hammering the Abdomen and Chest with the Large Round Pestle

Repeat all of the steps on pages 119–23 above, using the hammer and the large round pestle to treat the area around the navel, the upper abdomen, and the chest (fig. 6.14).

Repeating the tapping steps with the large pestle improves circulation because the pressure from the treatment radiates over a wider circumference.

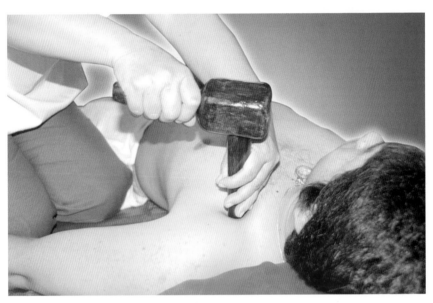

Fig. 6.14. Hammering the chest with the large round pestle

Treating Problems of the Arm and Hand, Supine Position

Common problems: Arm pain usually results from muscle spasm and tightness, which can arise from many factors including repetitive strain and overexertion during carrying, lifting, etc. Pain may be accompanied by numbness, tingling, or restricted range of motion in the shoulder, elbow, or hand.

1. Have your student press her palm against your hand as you provide resistance. This pushing makes the tendon in the shoulder taut, which reveals any problems more easily. With your other hand, palpate the shoulder region.
2. Move your resistance hand around so that your student presses in a variety of directions—up, down, to the side, etc.—as you continue to palpate the shoulder.

✿ Hammering the Inner Arm

As a general rule, you will use the larger round pestle for muscles and the smaller pestle for tendons. Beginning at the shoulder, tap and slide along the midline of the inside of the arm (fig. 6.15).

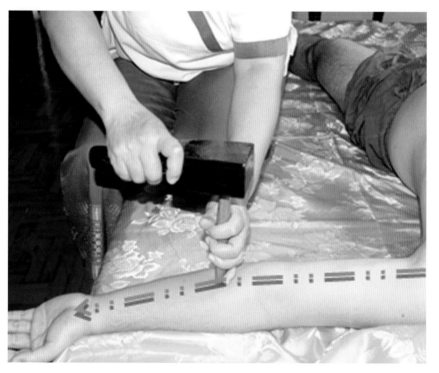

Fig. 6.15. Tap gently as you slide the pestle down the inner arm.

❂ Hammering the Hand

1. With the palm facing up, hammer down the muscles of the palm and into the pinkie finger (fig. 6.16). It is essential to be gentle and careful, tapping alongside the bones of the finger, not directly on them.

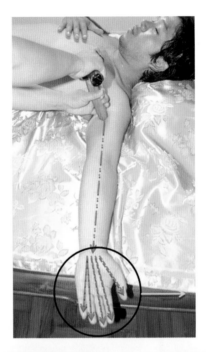

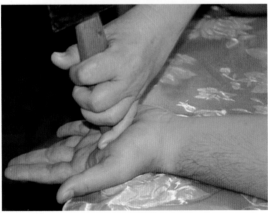

Fig. 6.16. Treating the palm

2. Next, hammer down the palm and the ring finger (again, working beside the bones rather than on them).

3. Repeat this step 3 more times, hammering into the middle finger, index finger, and thumb.

4. Next, turn the student's arm and hand over, and repeat steps 1–3 on the back of the hand (fig. 6.17).

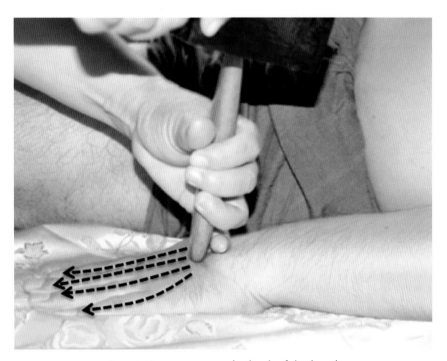

Fig. 6.17. Hammering the back of the hand

◕ Hammering the Outer Arm and Elbow

1. Beginning at the shoulder, tap down along the front of the arm to the wrist (see fig. 6.18 on page 128).

2. To work on the elbow, hammer on the fleshy part of the muscles, angling and sliding toward the bony olecranon of the ulna. Do not tap directly on the bone (see fig. 6.19 on page 128).

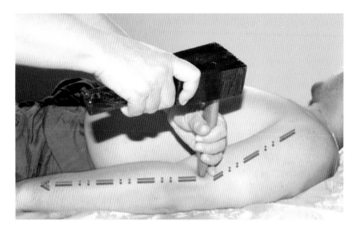

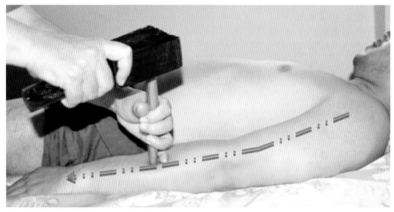

Fig. 6.18. Hammering the outer arm

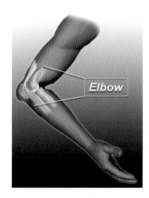

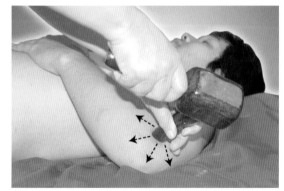

Fig. 6.19. Hammering the elbow

Hammering the Groin Area, Supine Position

The groin area is both significant and delicate. The practitioner should always be cautious, gentle, and respectful in treating this region. The correct positions for the individual receiving the treatment are shown. The hammering or tapping here, as elsewhere, releases energy that is that is stuck.

1. Begin by hammering around the hip bone, taking care to hammer away from the bone rather than on it.
2. Next, move to the pelvic region, angling and sliding the pestle from the center outward (fig. 6.20). Be careful not to hammer against the pubic or pelvic bones.

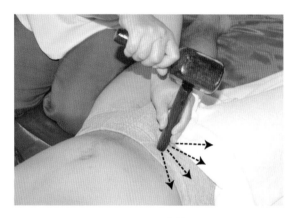

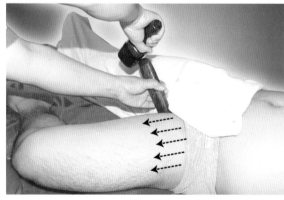

Fig. 6.20.
Hammering the groin

Treatment of the Legs and Feet, Supine Position

Common problems: Leg pain, knee pain, low back pain, knee swelling, patella disclocation, muscle strain, ankle sprain.

Before beginning work on the legs, it is best to stretch them out and relax them a little bit. This can be done simply by bending the knee upward and then putting the leg down flat a few times. This body management can help alleviate leg pain as well as back pain because of the close connection between the lower body and the back.

It should be kept in mind that many problems in the back actually derive from the legs, which can change the position of the spine. Tok Sen helps loosen and relax the muscles and tendons in the leg so that they can perform their function in a more natural fashion without distorting the spine.

Hammering the Thigh

When working on the thigh, you will first be hammering and sliding downward along each significant meridian or Sen line, then working across it.

It is helpful to use the larger pestle for the big muscles of the thigh and a smaller pestle for the tendons.

1. While keeping the whole leg on the floor or table, bend the knee to about a 90-degree angle (fig. 6.21).
2. Hammer down the outside of the thigh from the hip to the knee, then downward across sections of this line several times, from the front to the back of the leg.
3. Repeat step 2 down the top of the thigh, then repeat it again on the inside of the thigh (see fig. 6.22 on page 132). The sliding motion can be assisted by applying a small amount of oil to the area.

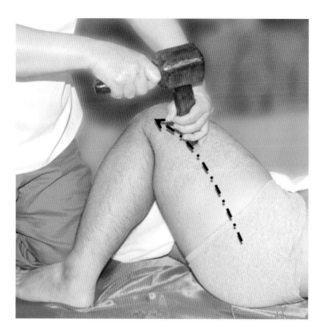

First, hammer down the outer thigh from hip to knee. Then hammer downward several times along this line from the front of the leg to the back.

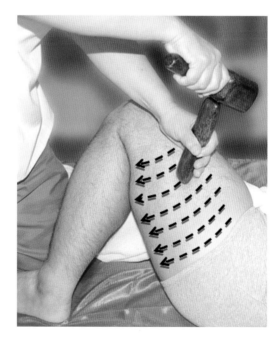

Fig. 6.21. Hammering the outer thigh

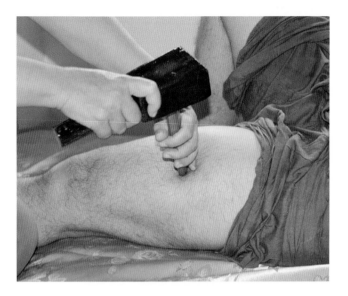

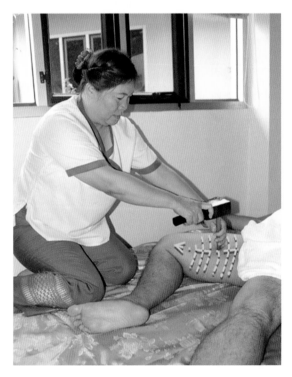

Fig. 6.22. Hammering the front and inner portions of the thigh

✿ *Hammering the Knee*

Straighten the leg so that the knee faces upward, and place a small pillow beneath it, to support the knee in a partially bent position.

1. Tap all around the kneecap, always sliding outward from it (fig. 6.23).
2. Use the four-legged pestle to tap all around the patellar tendon (fig. 6.24).

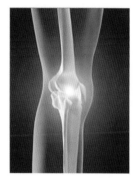
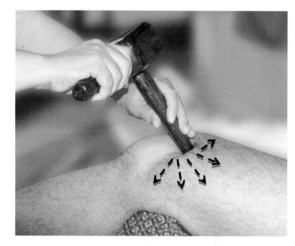

Fig. 6.23. Tapping around the kneecap

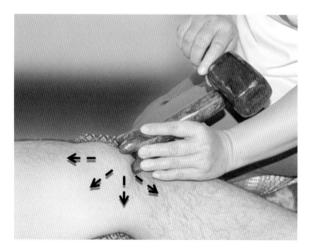

Fig. 6.24. Using the four-legged pestle to tap the patellar tendon

☀ Hammering the Lower Leg

1. Tap from the knee down to the ankle along several lines, being careful not to tap on the bone (fig. 6.25).
2. Following the shinbone down along the inside of the leg, tap outward/horizontally from the shin bone into the muscle belly along several short lines.
3. Next, tap in vertical lines down the inside of the calf to the ankle (fig. 6.26).
4. Next, use the two-legged pestle to tap down along both sides of the tibia simultaneously.

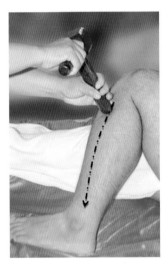

Fig. 6.25. Hammering outer calf

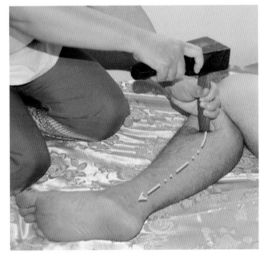

Fig. 6.26. Hammering the inner calf

✿ Hammering the Foot

Before working on the foot, the practitioner should determine the appropriate areas for treatment by feeling and lightly squeezing the ankle and foot. The four-legged pestle can be used for the bottom of the shin bone and the malleolus, as well for any other areas that would benefit from treatment on both sides.

1. Use the small wedge to treat the top of the foot down to the toes (fig. 6.27).
2. Use the four-legged pestle to treat the top of the foot and the outer ankle bone as shown in figure 6.28.

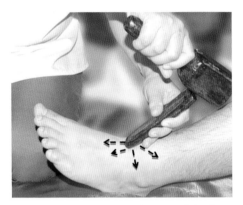

Fig. 6.27. Hammering the top of the foot

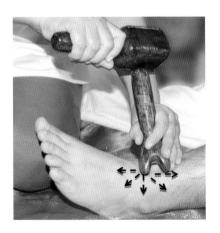 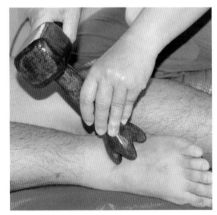

Fig. 6.28. Hammering the foot with the four-legged pestle

TREATING THE BACK OF THE BODY, PRONE POSITION

The prone position is useful for hammering the entire area of the back and legs (fig. 6.29). This includes all the major muscles groups and the significant lines on the posterior portion of the body. It also extends down to the calf, hamstrings and Achilles tendons, and soles.

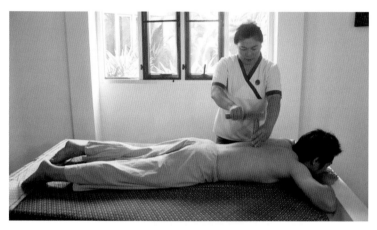

Fig. 6.29. The prone position

⟳ Treating the Spine with Tok Sen

The spinal cord is crucial to proper function and mobility, such that even minor disturbances to its structure can cause numbness, pain, dysfunction, and disability. It should be immediately noted that the practitioner never hammers directly on the spine. However, if care is

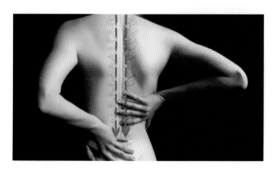

Fig. 6.30. Treating spinal problems

exercised, Tok Sen treatment can greatly assist in relieving many of the problems associated with the spine.

⚙ Hammering the Paravertebral Muscles

Common problems: Paravertebral spasms, tightness, and restricted range of motion in the trunk. Often these symptoms are caused by inflammation or protrusion of the intervertebral discs, which then put pressure on the muscles and tendons.

1. First, using the two-legged pestle, hammer the muscles that run vertically along each side of the thoracic spine, taking care not to hammer on the spine itself (fig. 6.31). Start at the top of the thoracic region and hammer down to the lumbar region. Tap up and down 10 times.

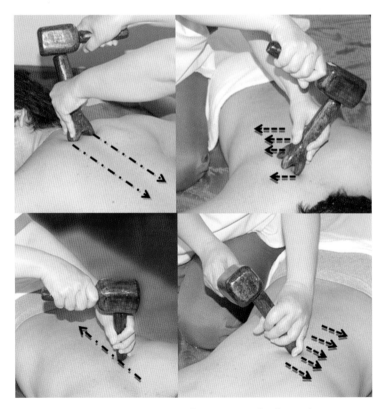

Fig. 6.31. Hammering the paravertebral muscles

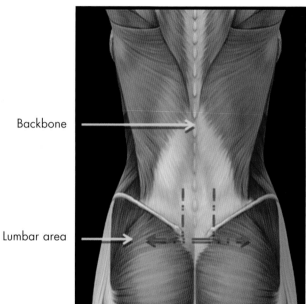

Backbone

Lumbar area

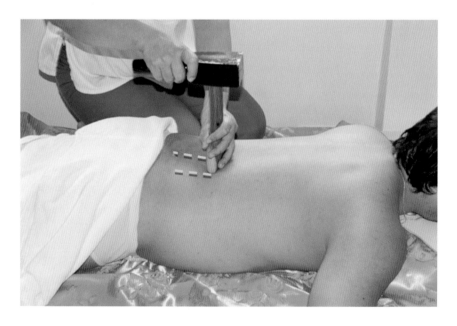

Fig. 6.32. Hammer vertically up and down the lumbar area

Note: If the two-legged pestle is too narrow to span the spine without touching it, use a single pestle and tap each side separately.

2. Next, hammer each of these spinal lines outward, moving downward in sections, and tapping and sliding away from the spine in each section. Doing this properly results in the easing of stiffness and pain not just in the back but also in other regions of the body.

✲ Hammering the Lumbar Region

Common problems: Lumbar strain and pain, spinal cord inflammation.

Pain, rigidity, and other problems can be located in the lower back because of stress, heavy lifting, or strains. Thorough treatment of the lumbar area relieves pain and can even assist with problems such as spondylolisthesis (forward displacement of vertebra), though such treatment should only be undertaken by a highly trained Tok Sen practitioner.

1. Using a single pestle, hammer 10 times up and down the muscles that run vertically on either side of the lumbar spine (fig. 6.32). Muscles will loosen and relax.
2. At the base of the lumbar spine, hammer away from the spine on either side out to the edge of the back (fig. 6.33).

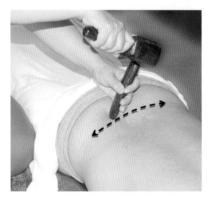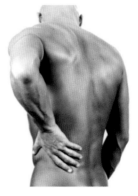

Fig. 6.33. Hammering the base of the lumbar region

☯ Hammering the Coccyx

The next area treated is the coccyx, or tailbone. The practitioner should palpate the area carefully to determine whether there are problems emanating from the coccyx.

Tap away from the coccyx on either side as shown in figure 6.34.

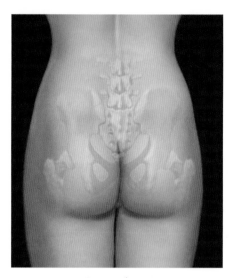

Coccyx bone

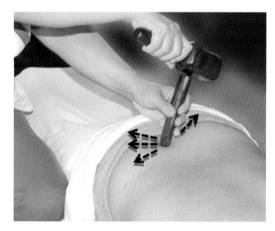

Fig. 6.34. Hammering the coccyx

⟁ Treating Backs of the Legs and Feet

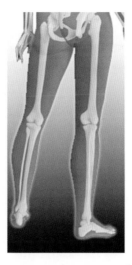

Fig. 6.35. The posterior leg

⟁ *Hammering the Back of the Thigh*

1. Tap and slide downward along the center of the back of the thigh, moving slowly from the upper thigh to the back of the knee (fig. 6.36).
2. Tap and slide outward from this central line in both directions, covering the whole back of the thigh in sections.

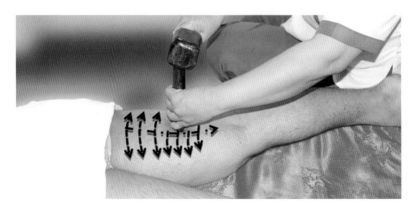

Fig. 6.36. Hammering the back of thigh

☯ Hammering the Back of the Knee

Using the larger pestle, tap downward in sections against the back of the knee (fig. 6.37).

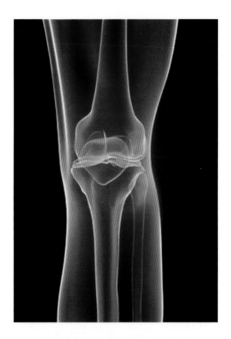

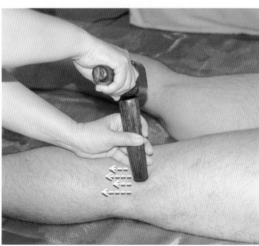

Fig. 6.37. Hammering the back of the knee

⟳ *Hammering the Sole of the Foot*

Before hammering, palpate the bottom of the foot to locate the large tendons extending in to each toe, as shown in figure 6.38a. Then hammer in straight lines from the heel along the sole and into each toe (fig. 6.38b).

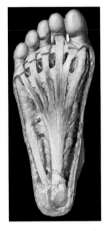
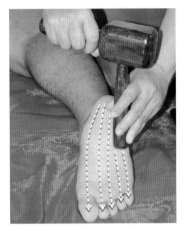

a   b

Fig. 6.38. Hammering the tendons on the sole of the foot

TREATMENT IN THE SIDE-LYING POSITION

A side-lying position can be helpful in treating ailments of the neck, shoulder, side of the ribcage, hip, sciatic nerve, calf muscles, and others (fig. 6.39). While the fundamental treatment and principles of the side-lying position are the same as for the other positions, some variations are needed.

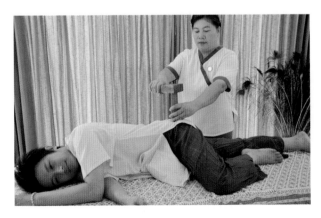

Fig. 6.39. Side-lying position

🌀 Hammering the Side of the Body

To begin, the patient should do a few light stretches against resistance to relax and highlight the tendons of the shoulder and hip.

🌀 *Warm-Up Stretches*

1. Lying on his side, the client should partially bend the top leg at the knee.
2. The practitioner should place one hand on top of the client's knee and apply resistance as the client rotates his hip and raises the knee up. The practitioner's other hand should be on the client's hip, in order to feel the tendons there.
3. Repeat steps 2 and 3 with the arm instead of the leg. The practitioner should apply resistance at the elbow while palpating the shoulder with the other hand. The client should raise his arm.

🌀 *Hammering the Neck, Side-Lying Position*

Use a small pillow to support the client's head, if desired.

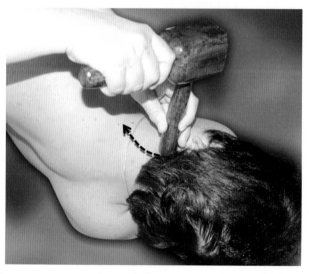

Fig. 6.40. Treating the neck: hammering the side of the neck

1. Gently hold the head with one hand while palpating the side of the neck with the other hand.
2. Lightly tap downward along the side of the neck as shown in figure 6.40.
3. Tap the upper border of the shoulder blade, moving outward in several directions as shown in fig. 6.41.

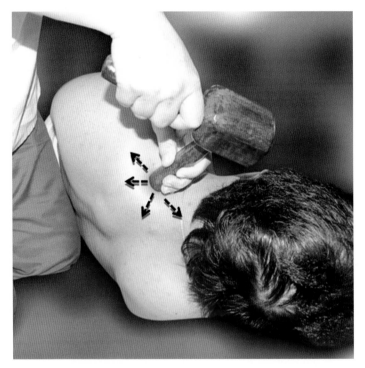

Fig. 6.41. Treating neck: hammering the upper border of the scapula

◉ Hammering the Torso, Side-Lying Position

Treatment in the side position is similar to prone, but the hammering is done on one side of the spine only.

1. Hammer one line down the middle of the back, from the shoulder to the lumbar vertebrae.
2. Hammer transversely toward this line in several places.

☯ Hammering at the Lower Back and Hip, Side-Lying Position

1. Hammer alongside one side of the lumbar spine as shown in figure 6.42. Note that you should hammer only the side that is closest to you.

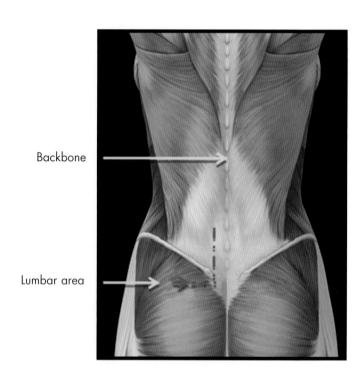

Backbone

Lumbar area

Fig. 6.42. Treating the lumbar spine

2. Hammer in a transverse line from the hip to the bottom of the lumbar spine.
3. Hammer and slide downward along the hip as shown in figure 6.43. Nerves that are stuck in this region need to be freed so that the energy can flow properly. Avoid hitting on the bone while trying to release nerves that are caught.
4. Palpate frequently to determine where the treatment should be continued.

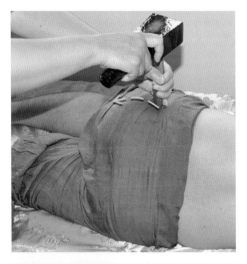

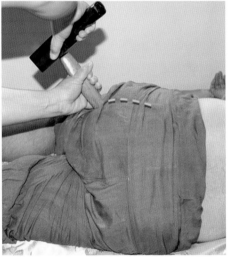

Fig. 6.43. Hammering the hip area

🌀 Hammering the Leg, Side-Lying Position

1. Tap downward along the side of the leg as shown in figure 6.44 on page 148.
2. Then tap outward from this line toward the front and the back of the thigh.
3. Tap and slide along the lower leg, from the knee to the ankle, as shown in figure 6.45a on page 148.

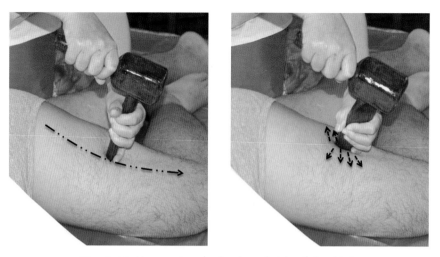

Fig. 6.44. Hammering the back and side of the thigh

4. Tap around the head of the fibula (fig. 6.45b).
5. Palpate the lower leg as the client flexes his knee, then tap any other areas that feel constricted. Tap and slide from the back of the fibula toward the muscles of the calf, as shown in figure 6.45c.

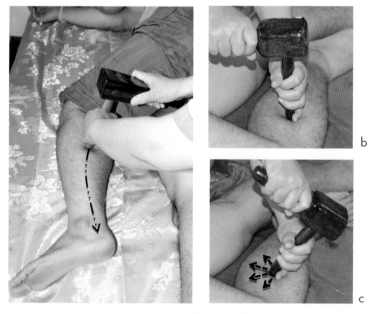

Fig. 6.45. Hammering the side of the calf

🌀 *Treating the Ankle, Side-Lying Position*

Use the four-legged pestle, or the pestle of your choice, to tap around the ankle bone, releasing nerves and tendons that are caught (fig. 6.46). Remember to hammer in a direction away from the anklebone itself.

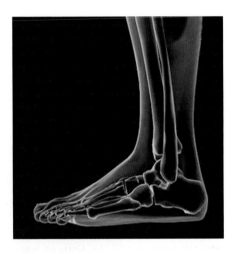

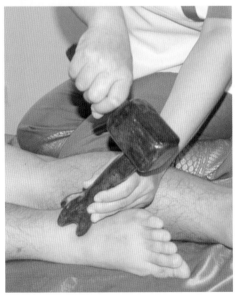

Fig. 6.46. Hammering the ankle with the four-legged pestle

TREATMENT IN THE SITTING POSITION

The sitting position is best for treating ailments of the neck and back, including muscle tension and migraine pain. Note, however, that tapping on the neck also sends vibrations to the brain, so this tapping should be done very lightly.

 ## Hammering in the Sitting Position

Begin by hammering downward alongside the spine, from the neck to the lumbar vertebrae (fig. 6.47). Tap and slide down one side first; then repeat on the other side.

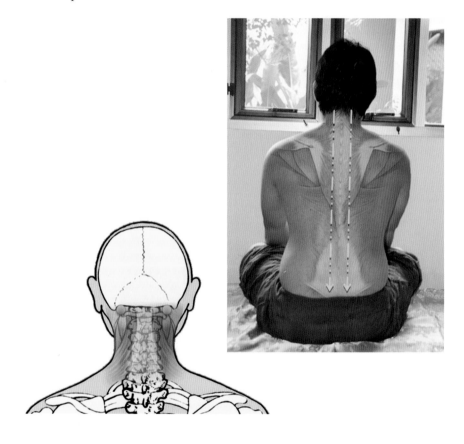

Fig. 6.47. Tok Sen treatment in the sitting position

⊘ Hammering the Neck, Sitting Position

Common problems: Poor posture, overexertion, eye strain, migraine, stiff neck.

1. Locate the main tendons of the neck and hammer up and down each side ten times (fig. 6.48a).
2. Palpate around the occipital bone, then hammer downward and outward from it as needed, as shown in figue 6.48b.
3. Tap and slide down the sides of the neck as shown in figure 6.48c.

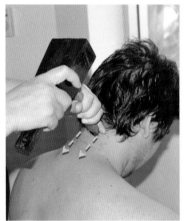

a

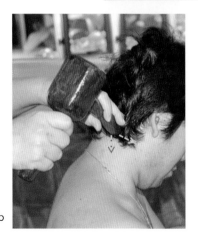

b

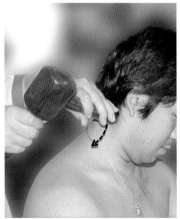

c

Fig. 6.47. Hammering the neck

⊘ Treating the Shoulders, Sitting Position

After treating the neck, the Tok Sen practitioner can move out to the shoulders. Treatment of the shoulders should include the top part of the shoulder as well as the upper back between the shoulder blades. Treating this region is especially effective for issues that have developed from heavy lifting.

1. Beginning beside the lower cervical vertebrae, tap and slide from the spine outward along the top of the shoulder (fig. 6.49).
2. Tap one or two lines this way, until you reach the upper border of the scapula.
3. Tap and slide down along the inner border of the scapula (fig. 6.50), then tap and slide in short horizontal strokes from the scapula border toward the spine.

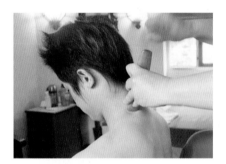 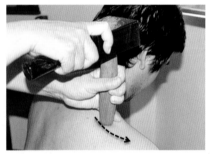

Fig. 6.49. Hammering the upper border of the shoulder

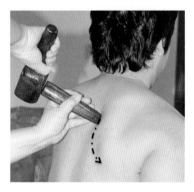 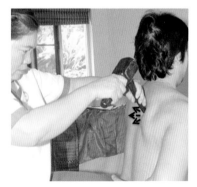

Fig. 6.50. Hammering the inner border of the shoulder blade

TREATMENT ACCORDING TO THE AFFECTED
AREA OF THE BODY

AREA OF BODY	POSSIBLE SYMPTOMS	SUGGESTED TREATMENT
Head and neck	Headache and migraine, neck pain, stiff neck, dizziness, eye problems caused by neck tension	Hammer both neck tendons up and down 10 times.
Shoulder	Shoulder sprain from working too hard or carrying heavy loads	Hammer both shoulder tendons up and down 10 times.
Back	Paravertebral pain and tightness, limited range of trunk motion caused by tendon compresion and spinal cord inflammation	Hammer paravertebral muscles from neck to the lumbars up and down 10 times.
Lower back	Low back pain, lumbar sprain, limited range of trunk motion, spondylolithesis	Hammer at lumbar area.
Thigh	Thigh pain with lumbar pain, thigh muscle tightness caused by falling, compressed sacrum, walking difficulties	Hammer lumbar area on both sides, and hamstring area (back of thigh).
Knee	Knee pain, knee swelling caused by patella dislocation, muscle tightness, difficulty walking	Hammer around patella, around patellar tendon, popliteal area, calf tendon to Achilles tendon.
Arm and hand	Arm pain, shoulder pain and shoulder dislocation, cannot move arm, hand pain or numbness	Hammer at shoulder tendon on lateral and medial sides, wrist, both sides of hand.

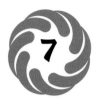

Meridian Detoxification Therapy

The tissues and meridians of the body are subject to a build-up of toxins, which can interfere with muscle and tendon flexibility and with the functioning of the organs. Removing toxins from the body is therefore an important element in traditional healing. Generally, toxins can be removed in only a small number of ways: via cleansing the organs—leading to excretions from the bladder and bowels—and via the skin, which is the body's biggest organ.

On the following pages, you will find information about three powerful methods of skin detoxification that are popular treatments throughout Asia: skin detoxification massage, cupping therapy, and Gua Sha.*

SKIN DETOXIFICATION MASSAGE

By massaging the abdomen in specific ways, a knowledgeable practitioner can prompt the internal organs to "dump" toxic deposits.

For general detoxification, you can massage the abdomen in clockwise spirals, working outward from the navel, as shown in figure 7.1. In

---

*For information on detoxification via the bladder and bowels, see Mantak Chia and William U. Wei, *Cosmic Detox* (Rochester, Vt.: Destiny Books, 2005).

this process, you will be gently squeezing toxins out from the internal organs. Figure 7.2 shows the relationship of the internal organs to the different sections of the abdomen. For more detailed massage detoxification practices, see the first volume in this series, *Chi Nei Tsang*.*

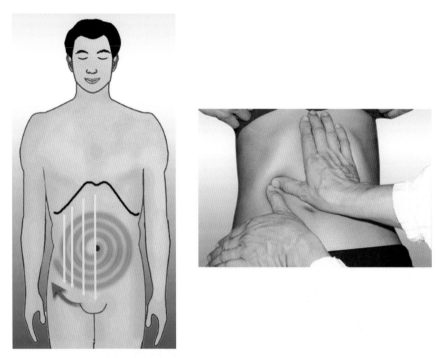

Fig. 7.1. Massaging the abdomen for detoxification

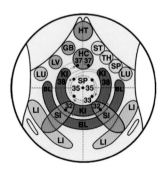

Fig. 7.2. The organ areas of the abdomen

---

*Mantak Chia, *Chi Nei Tsang* (Rochester, Vt.: Destiny Books, 2005), 160–97.

CUPPING THERAPY

Cupping therapy is used to cleanse and detoxify the body by pulling built-up impurities from deep in the body out through the skin. The technique relies on suction, which is created in specially designed glass or plastic cups that are placed in key positions on the body (fig. 7.3). When suction is created via a pump or controlled flame, the skin pulls up into the cup, drawing toxins outward. This treatment can be used on its own or in conjunction with an overall treatment plan of massage and Chinese medicine.

The cupping equipment presented in figure 7.4 is more modern than the traditional glass cups, which rely on flame to create suction, but the strategy, philosophy, and goals are the same. The procedure is easy but practical. Essentially, toxins and contaminated blood are removed from the body.

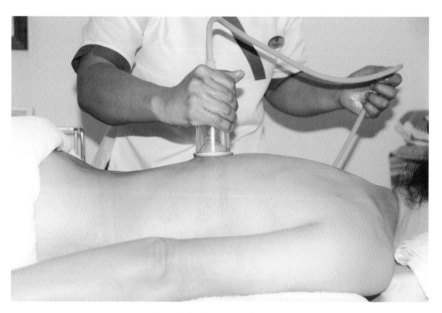

Fig. 7.3. Cupping therapy

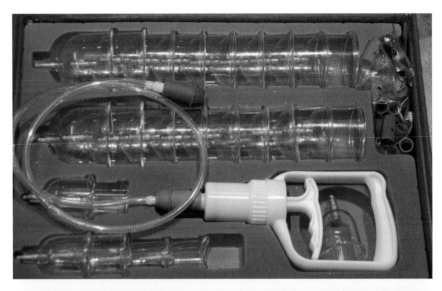

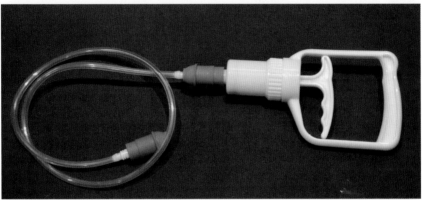

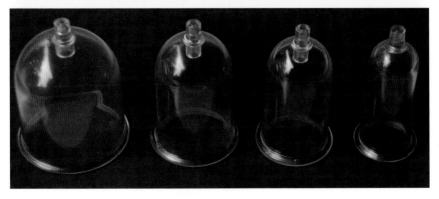

Fig. 7.4. Cupping tools

Cupping along the Spine for Detoxification

This treatment begins with the cups set beside the seventh cervical vertebra, which can be located as follows.

Locating the Seventh Cervical Vertebra

1. With the patient lying prone, place the fingers of one hand gently on the vertebrae at the back of the neck.
2. Have your patient gently raise her head as you palpate the vertebrae of the neck. C7 will be the vertebra that recedes or "disappears" from under your finger as the head is raised.
3. You can have the patient raise and lower her head 2 to 3 times to be sure of the point.

Setting the Cups

1. Using the C7 vertebra as a landmark, count down one more vertebra to T1. On both sides of T1, approximately 1.5 finger-widths from the spine, is the acupuncture point Urinary Bladder 11, which lies over the lungs.
2. Set one cup on each side of the spine, approximately over the UB11 point. By palpation, this point will be about the same level as the upper border of the scapula; however, you will want to place the cups between the scapula and the spine.
3. Pump the suction pump 3 times. Notice the skin drawing upward inside the cup.
4. Repeat steps 2 and 3 several more times, setting cups in two vertical rows on the Urinary Bladder meridian, alongside the spine. Leave about an inch below each cup before you set the next one. Do not continue below the level between L2 and L3 (UB23), which is the point corresponding to the kidneys.

Each of the acupuncture points alongside the spine corresponds to a particular organ, as shown in figure 7.5. Cupping over these organ points helps to draw toxins from the organs themselves. Note, however, that you will have fewer cups than there are points; each cup will cover 2–3 points, depending on its size and the size of the patient.

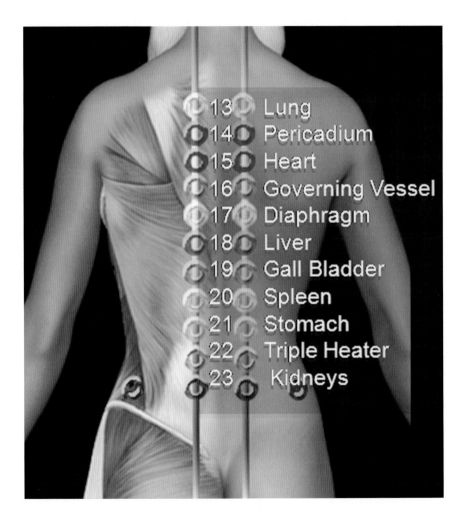

13 Lung
14 Pericadium
15 Heart
16 Governing Vessel
17 Diaphragm
18 Liver
19 Gall Bladder
20 Spleen
21 Stomach
22 Triple Heater
23 Kidneys

Fig. 7.5. Urinary Bladder meridian points along the spine
and their relationship to the organs

☯ *Removing the Cups*

5. Keep the cups on the body for 10–15 minutes. You will notice that the skin inside the cups will begin to darken during this time, which is a sign of the toxins moving outward.
6. To remove the cups, break the suction by gently pressing one finger into the skin just outside the cup. Slowly press your finger under the edge of the cup until the suction breaks: then it is safe to remove the cup.
7. This procedure sucks out toxins from the body; the darker the bruise, the more toxins have been released from inside the body.
8. Be sure to clean the cups thoroughly with alcohol or hot soapy water immediately after the session.

Meridian detox cupping therapy is an effective treatment for increasing energy and purifying the body. It permits energy to flow more freely and effectively, thus improving movement and reducing pain that may be lodged in different regions. It can be effective for many issues from the common cold to lung infections and other internal diseases. Furthermore, it is helpful with the joints and troubles such as back spasms or pain.

GUA SHA

Gua Sha removes pathogenic blood stagnation, promoting normal circulation and metabolic processes. It is valuable in the prevention and treatment of acute infectious illness, upper respiratory and digestive problems, and many other acute or chronic disorders.

The name *Gua Sha* is comprised of the two Chinese characters: *Gua*, meaning to scrape or rub, and *Sha* meaning sand. This name indicates both the action and the visual result of the practice. Gua Sha includes scraping the skin with the rounded edge of an instrument to encourage the formation of red spots—known as petechiae—on the surface of the skin.

Once these spots or *Sha* have been raised, the patient will experience immediate relief from pain, stiffness, fever, chill, cough, nausea, and so on. Like the cupping bruises, areas of Sha are direct evidence of toxins coming to the surface, and of stagnant blood moving once again. They will fade in two to thre days.

Gua Sha Tools

Gua Sha tools are traditionally made from horn (fig. 7.6), though modern practitioners use tools of many materials. The tools come in

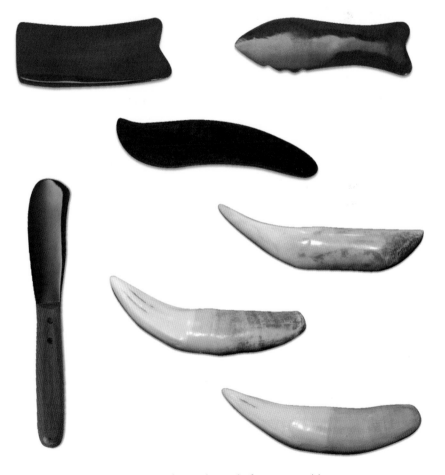

Fig. 7.6. Gua Sha tools made from natural horn

a variety of shapes and sizes, because different areas of the body—and different bodies—will require different approaches.

Gua Sha Scraping Technique

The scraping technique should be done in a systematic fashion. The angle and pressure applied needs to be correct for a proper treatment. Essentially this means that there are three main things to keep in mind:

1. **45-degree angle:** the Gua Sha tool should be held at a 45-degree angle from the surface of the skin (fig. 7.7).
2. **Even force:** an even amount of pressure should be maintained through each stroke: do not increase or reduce your pressure as you go.
3. **Uniform speed:** try to maintain a relatively slow, even speed throughout the treatment. Strokes that are too fast and/or too hard will cause tension and pain in the patient.

Oil should be applied to the area before the scraping begins. During scraping, the force must be even and appropriate, with no sudden change of speed or strength; scrape until red patches appear on the skin.

Gua Sha Therapy

Gua Sha can be applied to many parts of the body, including the back, neck, face, arms, legs, etc. (see fig. 7.8 on page 164) It can be used to relieve pain or other symptoms in a particular area of the body, and, because it releases blood stagnation, it can also be used for general health.

It is appropriate to scrape along bones and along muscles and connective tissue. However, remember to use less pressure against the bones, as they will be much more sensitive.

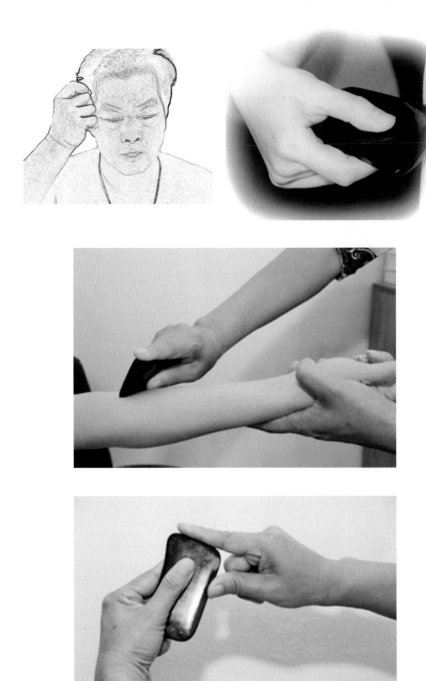

Fig. 7.7. Scraping technique

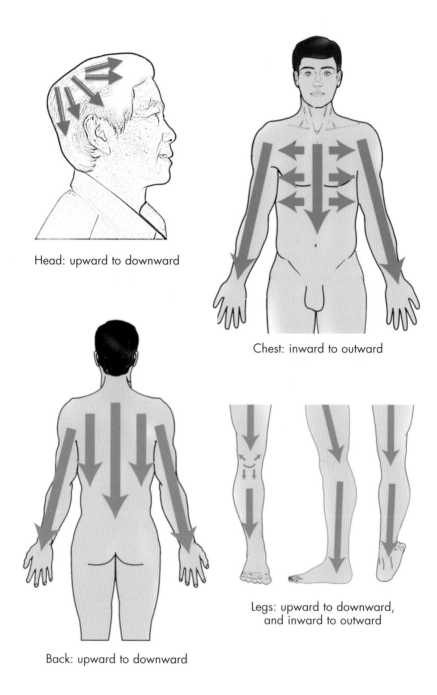

Head: upward to downward

Chest: inward to outward

Back: upward to downward

Legs: upward to downward, and inward to outward

Fig. 7.8. Gua Sha scraping directions

In addition, keep the following principles in mind:

- The sharp edge of the Gua Sha tool should be used for the joint areas between the bones.
- The surface to be scraped should be extended as much as possible.
- The torso, face, and limbs are to be scraped from the inside to the outside, and from the top toward the bottom.

Gua Sha Therapy on the Back

The exercise below details Gua Sha treatment on the upper back, which is a powerful treatment for common cold and other respiratory ailments. It also benefits the heart by improving circulation and alleviates conditions aggravated by tension in the muscles of the neck and upper back.

1. With your patient sitting or lying prone, perform some light massage on the area to be treated.
2. Apply a generous amount of oil, but not so much that it drips.
3. With the Gua Sha tool in your dominant hand, and your other hand resting gently on the patient's shoulder or back of the head, place the edge of the tool at the top of the spine, at a 45-degree angle to skin (see fig. 7.9 on page 166).
4. Press the tool gently into the skin and slide it downward along the spine. Use enough pressure to press the skin without causing pain, and maintain this pressure for the length of your stroke.
5. Repeat this same stroke 2 or 3 times in the same place, until you see redness or small spots appear. Do not press too hard or slide too fast; have your patient let you know if he is uncomfortable.
6. Next, repeat this scraping stroke down along the sides of the spine. Repeat each stroke a few times in the same place, until you see the petechiae, or until the area gets red.
7. Scrape downward in several lines along the back, and scrape outward across the shoulders.

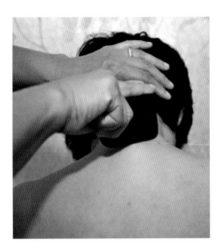

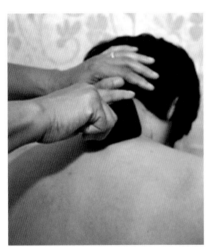 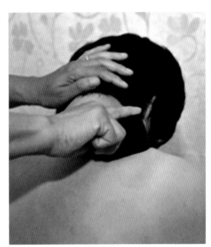

Fig. 7.9. Beginning Gua Sha treatment on the upper back

After Gua Sha, have the patient drink warm water to aid in metabolism. He may be achy in the treatment area for 2–3 days, which is normal. Patients should avoid exposing the treated area to cold or windy conditions.

The areas where Sha develops reveal underlying problems. From an organ perspective, more Sha in the upper back reveals stagnation around the heart and lungs, whereas more Sha in the mid-back can suggest stagnation of the liver, gallbladder, and spleen (fig. 7.10).

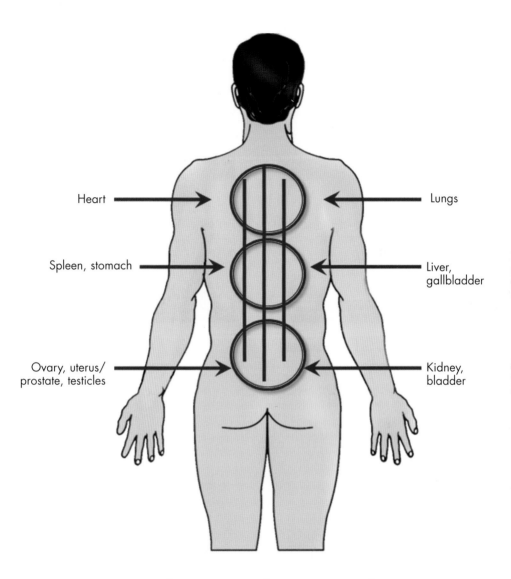

Heart

Lungs

Spleen, stomach

Liver,
gallbladder

Ovary, uterus/
prostate, testicles

Kidney,
bladder

Fig. 7.10. Areas of symptoms can indicate stagnation in the organs.

The figures on page 168 show some common Sha patterns on the back after treatment. An experienced practitioner can "read" these patterns and make recommendations for correcting internal imbalances.

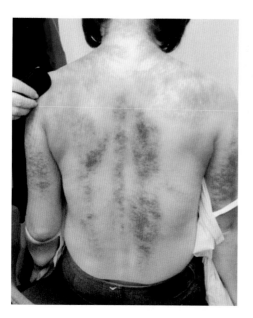

Fig. 7.11. Large red spots indicate an acidic body.

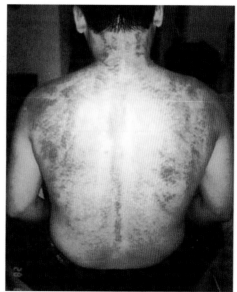

Fig. 7.12. Red flower spots reveal irregular blood circulation.

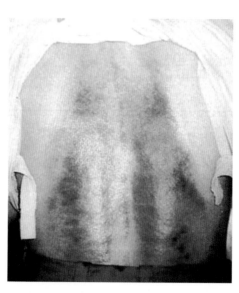

Fig. 7.13. Bluish black spots indicate toxins in the body.

Gua Sha Hand Reflexology

Figure 7.14 shows Gua Sha being applied to the hand. The hand is an excellent place to apply the principles of reflexology, which recognizes the hand as a mirror of the whole body. For example, the thumb and little finger correspond to the legs, the index and ring fingers the arms, and the middle finger the spine. Pain in a specific area is generally associated with a nodule or bump on the skin in a relevant position. These principles, which aim to treat pain or disease, are in addition to the overall health benefits of Gua Sha therapy.

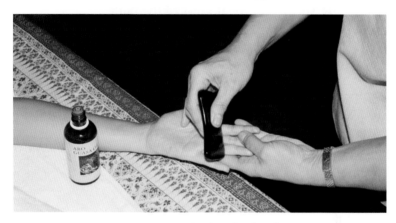

Fig. 7.14. Gua Sha hand reflexology

Gua Sha Facial Therapy

Gua Sha can be applied to the face, as shown in figure 7.15 below. Be sure to discuss the Gua Sha bruises—which will last for 2–3 days—with your patient before the treatment, and be sure to receive consent.

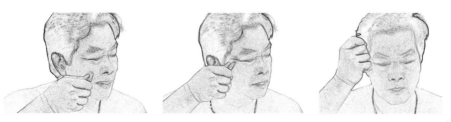

Fig. 7.15. Facial Gua Sha

Three Easy Benefits

Three main benefits of Gua Sha are: comfort, maintenance health care, and disease treatment.

1. **Gua Sha for comfort:** Enhances body strength and leaves you feeling fresh, vigorous, and energetic throughout the day.
2. **Gua Sha for health care:** Promotes blood circulation, which reduces pain associated with many health problems.
3. **Gua Sha for disease treatment:** Specific ailments can be treated with Gua Sha on pertinent areas of the body.

The cautions mentioned throughout the book relative to any healing or maintenance technique must always be at the forefront of a good practitioner's mind. While there is likely to be some pain and bruising resulting from the scraping, this should not last more than a few days.

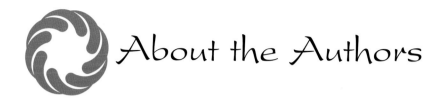 # About the Authors

MANTAK CHIA

Mantak Chia has been studying the Taoist approach to life since childhood. His mastery of this ancient knowledge, enhanced by his study of other disciplines, has resulted in the development of the Universal Healing Tao system, which is now being taught throughout the world.

Mantak Chia was born in Thailand to Chinese parents in 1944. When he was six years old, he learned from Buddhist monks how to sit and "still the mind." While in grammar school he learned traditional Thai boxing, and he soon went on to acquire considerable skill in aikido, yoga, and Tai Chi. His studies of the Taoist way of life began in earnest when he was a student in Hong Kong, ultimately leading to his mastery of a wide variety of esoteric disciplines, with the guidance of several masters, including Master I Yun, Master Meugi, Master Cheng Yao Lun, and Master Pan Yu. To better understand the mechanisms behind healing energy, he also studied Western anatomy and medical sciences.

Master Chia has taught his system of healing and energizing practices to tens of thousands of students and trained more than two thousand instructors and practitioners throughout the world. He has established centers for Taoist study and training in many countries around the globe. In June of 1990, he was honored by the International Congress of Chinese Medicine and Qi Gong (Chi Kung), which named him the Qi Gong Master of the Year.

WILLIAM U. WEI

Born after World War II, growing up in the Midwest area of the United States, and trained in Catholicism, William Wei became a student of the Tao under Master Mantak Chia in the early 1980s. In the later 1980s he became a senior instructor of the Universal Healing Tao, specializing in one-on-one training. In the early 1990s William Wei moved to Tao Garden, Thailand, and assisted Master Mantak Chia in building Tao Garden Taoist Training Center. For six years William traveled to over thirty countries, teaching with Master Mantak Chia and serving as marketing and construction coordinator for the Tao Garden. Upon completion of Tao Garden in December 2000, he became project manager for all the Universal Tao publications and products. With the purchase of a mountain with four waterfalls in southern Oregon, USA, in the late 1990s, William Wei is presently completing a Taoist Mountain Sanctuary for personal cultivation, higher-level practices, and ascension. William Wei is the coauthor with Master Chia of *Sexual Reflexology*, *Living in the Tao*, and the Taoist poetry book of 366 daily poems, *Emerald River*, which expresses the feeling, essence, and stillness of the Tao. He is also the cocreator with Master Mantak Chia of the Universal Healing Tao Chi Cards, upon which this book has been based, under the pen name The Professor—Master of Nothingness, the Myth that takes the Mystery out of Mysticism. William U. Wei, also known as Wei Tzu, is a pen name for this instructor so the instructor can remain anonymous and can continue to become a blade of grass in a field of grass.

The Universal Healing Tao System and Training Center

THE UNIVERSAL HEALING TAO SYSTEM

The ultimate goal of Taoist practice is to transcend physical boundaries through the development of the soul and the spirit within the human. That is also the guiding principle behind the Universal Healing Tao, a practical system of self-development that enables individuals to complete the harmonious evolution of their physical, mental, and spiritual bodies. Through a series of ancient Chinese meditative and internal energy exercises, the practitioner learns to increase physical energy, release tension, improve health, practice self-defense, and gain the ability to heal him- or herself and others. In the process of creating a solid foundation of health and well-being in the physical body, the practitioner also creates the basis for developing his or her spiritual potential by learning to tap into the natural energies of the sun, moon, earth, stars, and other environmental forces.

The Universal Healing Tao practices are derived from ancient techniques rooted in the processes of nature. They have been gathered and integrated into a coherent, accessible system for well-being that works directly with the life force, or chi, that flows through the meridian system of the body.

Master Chia has spent years developing and perfecting techniques for teaching these traditional practices to students around the world through ongoing classes, workshops, private instruction, and healing sessions, as well as books and video and audio products. Further information can be obtained at www.universal-tao.com.

THE UNIVERSAL HEALING TAO TRAINING CENTER

The Tao Garden Resort and Training Center in northern Thailand is the home of Master Chia and serves as the worldwide headquarters for Universal Healing Tao activities. This integrated wellness, holistic health, and training center is situated on eighty acres surrounded by the beautiful Himalayan foothills near the historic walled city of Chiang Mai. The serene setting includes flower and herb gardens ideal for meditation, open-air pavilions for practicing Chi Kung, and a health and fitness spa.

The center offers classes year round, as well as summer and winter retreats. It can accommodate two hundred students, and group leasing can be arranged. For information on courses, books, products, and other resources, see below.

RESOURCES

Universal Healing Tao Center
274 Moo 7, Luang Nua, Doi Saket, Chiang Mai, 50220 Thailand
Tel: (66)(53) 495-596 Fax: (66)(53) 495-852
E-mail: universaltao@universal-tao.com
Web site: www.universal-tao.com

For information on retreats and the health spa, contact:
Tao Garden Health Spa & Resort
E-mail: info@tao-garden.com, taogarden@hotmail.com
Web site: www.tao-garden.com

Good Chi • Good Heart • Good Intention

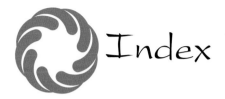 Index

Page numbers in *italics* refer to illustrations.

abdominal organs, 84–85, *85*
abdominal pain, 20, 21, 22, 28, 29
alcohol, 116
anatomy, Chinese medical, 30–31
   Gall Bladder meridian, 31–32, *32*
   Heart meridian, 38, *38*
   Kidney meridian, 41, *41*
   Large Intestine meridian, 35, *35*
   Liver meridian, 33, *33*
   Lung meridian, 34, *34*
   Pericardium meridian, 42, *42*
   Small Intestine meridian, 39, *39*
   Spleen meridian, 37, *37*
   Stomach meridian, 36–37, *36*
   Triple Heater meridian, 43, *43*
   Urinary Bladder meridian, 40–41, *41*
anatomy, Thai medical,15, 16–18, *17*
   descriptions of ten energy channels, 19–29, *20–29*
   names of ten energy channels, 18–19
   Sen 1: Itha, 19–20, *20*
   Sen 2: Pingkla, 21, *21*
   Sen 3: Summana, 22, *22*

Sen 4: Kanlataree, 23, *23*
Sen 5: Hadsarangsri, 24–25, *24*
Sen 6: Tawaree, 25, *25*
Sen 7: Jantapusank, 26, *26*
Sen 8: Rusum, 27, *27*
Sen 9: Sukumang, 28, *28*
Sen 10: Sikinee, 29, *29*
anatomy, Western medical
   fascia, 11–12, *12*
   ligaments, 11–12, *12*
   muscles, 6–9, *8–9*
   nerves and blood vessels, 13
   tendons, 10–11, *10*
anger, upper body and, 67
angina pectoris, 23
ankles, 104–5, *104–5*, 149, *149*
anterior hip, 96
appendicitis, 25
armor, 11, 59, 112
arms, 124–28, 153
arteries, 13
asthma, 22
aura, 56, 57

back pain, 20, 21
Belt Channel, 50

blockages, 110

blood circulation, 112

blood detoxification, 119

blood vessels, 13

body preparation, 46–49

Bone Marrow Breathing, 48

bronchitis, 22

Bubbling Spring point, 109, *109*

cervical spine, *14*, 77

channels, 12, 50

chest, 122–24, *122–24*

chest pain, 22, 23, 24, 26, 27, 118

chest swelling, 118

chi, 12

Chia, Mantak, 49

Chiang Mai, 110

chills, 20, 21

China, 16

Chi Nei Tsang, 155

circle wedge pestle, 114, *115*

circulation, 59, 112

circulatory system, 13

coccyx, *14*, 77, 140, *140*

colds, 20, 21, 22

Cosmic Nutrition, 49

coughs, 22, 26, 27

cupping therapy, 156–60, *156–57*, *159*

deafness, 26, 27

depressive psychosis, 24

diarrhea, 28, 29

digestion, 22, 23, 59

dizziness, 20, 21, 118

Door of Life, 77, 79

dry mouth, 118

ear diseases, 26, 27

elbow and lower arm massage, 68–70, *69–70*

elbow syndrome, 118

emotional preparation, 49–52

energy, 59

epilepsy, 23

eye pain, 20, 21, 24

facial paralysis, 24, 26, 27

facial therapy, 169, *169*

fascia, 11–12, *12*

feet, 106–9, *106*, *108–9*, 135, *135*, 143, *143*

female infertility, 28, 29

fevers, 20, 21, 24

finger press, 60

fingers, growing auras of, 57

five-element diet, 48–49

flat wedge pestle, 114, *115*

four-legged knocker, 114, *115*

Functional Channel, 50

Fusion of the Five Elements, 49

gallbladder, 21

Gall Bladder meridian, 31–32, *32*

gastrointestinal diseases, 25, 26, 27

genitals, 90–92, *91–92*

Governor Channel, 50

groin area, 129

grounding, 47, 52

Gua Sha, 160–70

   benefits of, 170

   scraping technique, 162–63, *162–63*

   therapy, 163–69, *164*, *166–69*

   tools for, 161–62, *161*

Hadsarangsri, 24–25, *24*
hammers, Tok Sen, 113–14, *113*
hand reflexology, 73, *73*, 169, *169*
hands, 70–73, *71–73*, 126–27, *127*,
    153
hand techniques, 59–60
headaches, 20, 21, 112, 153
head and neck massage, 61–63, *62–63*
Healing Hands, 51, 55–57
heart disease, 22, 23
Heart meridian, 38, *38*
herbal oil, 116
hernia, 23, 25, 28, 29
hips, 93–98, *93–96*, 146–47, *146–47*
hysteria, 23

iliopsoas muscle, 96–97, *96*
impotence, 28, 29
India, 16
indigestion, 23
infertility, 28, 29
inguinal ligaments, 90–92, *91–92*
Inner Smile, 51, 53–54
Inner Structure of Tai Chi, The, 47
inner thigh, 92, *92*
intestinal diseases, 20, 21
Iron Shirt Chi Kung, 47, 52
Itha, 19–20, *20*

Jantapusank, 26, *26*
jaundice, 25

Kanlataree, 23, *23*
Kidney meridian, 41, *41*
kidneys, 85
knees, 23, 100–103, *100–103*, 133,
    133, 142, *142*, 153

Lanna region, 110
Large Intestine meridian, 35, *35*
leg paralysis, 25
legs, 98–105, *98*, *100–105*, 134, *134*
ligaments, 11–12, *12*
liver, 21, 84
Liver meridian, 33, *33*
love, 52
lower back, 79, *79*, 113, 146, *146*,
    153
lumbar spine, *14*, 77, 113, 118, 139,
    139, 146, *146*, 153
Lung meridian, 34, *34*

mania, 24
meditation, 51
    Healing Hands, 55–57
    Inner Smile, 53–54
    Microcosmic Orbit, 54–55
menstruation, 28, 29
meridians, 12
    Gall Bladder, 31–32, *32*
    Heart, 38, *38*
    Kidney, 41, *41*
    Large Intestine, 35, *35*
    Liver, 33, *33*
    Lung, 34, *34*
    Pericardium, 42, *42*
    Small Intestine, 39, *39*
    Spleen, 37, *37*
    Stomach, 36–37, *36*
    Triple Heater, 43, *43*
    Urinary Bladder, 40–41, *40*
Microcosmic Orbit, 51, 52, 54–55
Ming Men, 77, 79
mobility, 59
muscles, 6–9, *8–9*

nasal obstruction, 20, 21

nausea, 22

navel, 82–84, *82–83*, 119–21, *120–21*

nerves, 13, 112

Nuad Thai

  genital area, 90–92, *91–92*

  hand techniques, 59–60

  head and neck, 61–63, *62–63*

  hips, 93–98, *93–96*

  legs, 98–105, *98, 100–105*

  Opening Stretch, 61

  psoas muscles, 86–90, *86–89*

  shoulder and upper arm, 64–67,
    64–67

  spine, 74–81, *74–76, 78–80*

  torso, 81–85, *81–83, 85*

  wrists and hands, 70–73, *71–73*

pain, 59, 112–13

palms, channeling force through,
  56

palpation, 117

paralysis, 24, *25*, 26, 27

paravertebral muscles, 137–39,
  137–38

patience, 117

Pericardium meridian, 42, *42*

peripheral nerves, 112

pestles, Tok Sen, 114–17, *115*

petechiae, 160–61, *168*

Pingkla, 21–22, *21–22*

piriformis, 95, *95*, 97–98, *98*

positioning, for Tok Sen, 116

posterior hip, 97

premature ejaculation, 28, 29

preparation

  emotional, 49–50

  energetic, 50–52

  physical, 46–49

psoas muscles, 75, *75*, 86–90, *86–89*

Rama III, King, 18

red spots, 160–61, *168*

reflexology, hand, 72, *73*, 169, *169*

ribcage, 81, *81*

Royal Traditional Thai Medicine Text,
  16

Rusum, 27, *27*

sacrum, *14*, 77

scapular pain, 118

schizophrenia, 23

scoop, 60

scraping technique, 162–63, *162–63*

Sen Sib, 16

  descriptions of, 19–29, *20–29*

  names of, 18–19

  Sen 1: Itha, 19–20, *20*

  Sen 2: Pingkla, 21, *21*

  Sen 3: Summana, 22, *22*

  Sen 4: Kanlataree, 23, *23*

  Sen 5: Hadsarangsri, 24–25, *24*

  Sen 6: Tawaree, 25, *25*

  Sen 7: Jantapusank, 26, *26*

  Sen 8: Rusum, 27, *27*

  Sen 9: Sukumang, 28, *28*

  Sen 10: Sikinee, 29, *29*

  starting points of on abdomen, *120*

shake, 60

shin problems, 118

shock, 23

shoulder and upper arm massage,
  64–67, *64–67*

shoulders, 20, 21, 112, 152, *152*, 153

sick energy, 51–52

Sikinee, 29, *29*

Simple Spinal Alignment, 15

sinusitis, 23

skin detoxification massage, 154–55, *155*

Small Intestine meridian, 39, *39*

spinal alignment, 15

spinal massage, 74–81, *74–76*, *78–80*

spine, 13–15, *14–15*, 76, 77, 158–60

spiral, 60

spleen, 85

Spleen meridian, 37, *37*

stagnant blood, 161

stagnation, 110

stiff neck, 20, 21, 118

Stomach meridian, 36–37, *36*

stress, 112

Sukumang, 28, *28*

surface sick energy, 51–52

Tai Chi Chi Kung, 47

tan tien, 85

Tao Yin exercises, 90

Tawaree, 25, *25*

tendinomuscular meridians, 30–31

   Gall Bladder, 31–32, *32*

   Heart, 38, *38*

   Kidney, 41, *41*

   Large Intestine, 35, *35*

   Liver, 33, *33*

   Lung, 34, *34*

   Pericardium, 42, *42*

   Small Intestine, 39, *39*

   Spleen, 37, *37*

   Stomach, 36–37, *36*

   Triple Heater, 43, *43*

   Urinary Bladder, 40–41, *41*

tendons, 10–11, *10*, 112

ten energy channels. *See* Sen Sib

Thailand, 110

Thai massage, 31

   benefits of, 58–59

   elbow and lower arm, 68–70, *69–70*

   genital area, 90–92, *91–92*

   hand techniques, 59–60

   head and neck, 61–63, *62–63*

   hips, 93–98, *93–96*

   legs, 98–105, *98*, *100–105*

   Opening Stretch, 61

   psoas muscles, 86–90, *86–89*

   shoulder and upper arm, 64–67, *64–67*

   spine, 74–81, *74–76*, *78–80*

   torso, 81–85, *81–83*, *85*

   wrists and hands, 70–73, *71–73*

   See also anatomy, Thai medical

thighs, 130–32, *131–32*, 141, *141*, 153

thoracic spine, *14*, 77

throat problems, 22, 24, 26, 27

Thrusting Channel, 50

tissues, 154

Tok Sen, 31

   benefits of, 112–13

   general guidelines for, 116–17

   overview of, 110–11

   prone position, 136–43

   protocols for ailments, 117–19, 153

   side-lying positions, 143–49

   sitting position, 150–52

supine position, 119–35
tools, *111*, 113–16, *113*, *115*
See also Tok Sen treatment
Tok Sen treatment
  ankles, 149, *149*
  arm and hand, 124–28, *125–28*
  chest, 122–24, *122–24*
  coccyx, 140, *140*
  foot, 135, *135*, 143, *143*
  groin area, 129, *129*
  hips, 146–47, *146–47*
  knee, 133, *133*, 142, *142*
  legs, 134, *134*, 147–48, *148*
  lumbar region, 139, *139*, 146,
    146
  navel, 119–21, *120–21*
  neck, 144–45, *144–45*, 151, *151*
  paravertebral muscles, 137–39,
    137–38
  shoulders, 152, *152*

thigh, 130–32, *131–32*, 141, *141*
  torso, 145, *145*
toothache, 24, 26, 27
torso, 81–85, *81–83*, 85
toxins, 154, 161
Triple Heater Meridian, 43, *43*
trunk tightness, 118
two-legged knocker, 114, *115*

Urinary Bladder meridian, 40–41, *41*
urinary tract, 20, 21
urination, 28, 29, 119
uterine bleeding, 28, 29

veins, 13
vertebrae, 76, 77

Wat Pho plaques, 18
wood, 113
wrists, 70–72, *71–72*

BOOKS OF RELATED INTEREST

Chi Nei Tsang
Chi Massage for the Vital Organs
by Mantak Chia

Advanced Chi Nei Tsang
Enhancing Chi Energy in the Vital Organs
by Mantak Chia

Chi Self-Massage
The Taoist Way of Rejuvenation
by Mantak Chia

Healing Light of the Tao
Foundational Practices to Awaken Chi Energy
by Mantak Chia

Healing Love through the Tao
Cultivating Female Sexual Energy
by Mantak Chia

Cosmic Detox
A Taoist Approach to Internal Cleansing
by Mantak Chia and William U. Wei

Simple Chi Kung
Exercises for Awakening the Life-Force Energy
by Mantak Chia and Lee Holden

Iron Shirt Chi Kung
by Mantak Chia

INNER TRADITIONS • BEAR & COMPANY
P.O. Box 388
Rochester, VT 05767
1-800-246-8648
www.InnerTraditions.com

Or contact your local bookseller